OXFORD MEDICAL PUBLICATIONS

Cardiothoracic
Critical Care

T0177916

Oxford Specialist Handbooks in Critical Care

Cardiothoracic Critical Care

Edited by

Robyn Smith
Department of Anaesthesia
Golden Jubilee National Hospital
Clydebank, UK

Mike Higgins
Golden Jubilee National Hospital
Clydebank, UK

Alistair Macfie
Department of Anaesthesia
Golden Jubilee National Hospital
Clydebank, UK

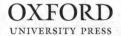

OXFORD
UNIVERSITY PRESS

OXFORD
UNIVERSITY PRESS

Great Clarendon Street, Oxford, OX2 6DP,
United Kingdom

Oxford University Press is a department of the University of Oxford.
It furthers the University's objective of excellence in research, scholarship,
and education by publishing worldwide. Oxford is a registered trade mark of
Oxford University Press in the UK and in certain other countries

Published in the United States of America by Oxford University Press
198 Madison Avenue, New York, NY 10016, United States of America

British Library Cataloguing in Publication Data

Data available

Library of Congress Control Number: 2013954327

ISBN 978-0-19-969295-8

Printed in Great Britain by
Ashford Colour Press Ltd, Gosport, Hampshire

Foreword

The specialty of intensive care is relatively new, starting in the 1950s with the polio epidemics, and maturing over the years to the point where it is now recognized as a specialty in its own right in the UK and several other countries worldwide.

Patients undergoing cardiac surgery have always been admitted directly to ICU post-operatively. Cardiothoracic intensive care, usually delivered by cardiothoracic anaesthetists, has resulted in excellent outcomes from major cardiac surgery. This system of patient care and its results are the envy of many other branches of surgery.

With developments in surgery, newer extracorporeal systems for support of cardiac and respiratory function, the survival of patients with congenital cardiac anomalies into adulthood and greater expectations from clinicians and patients, cardiothoracic intensive care is becoming a super-specialty of both intensive care medicine and anaesthesia. Indeed we are seeing the development of the cardiothoracic intensivist who is not also an anaesthetist.

The authors are established consultants in cardiothoracic anaesthesia and intensive care who bring many years of practical experience in the specialty to this handbook. Trainee attachments to cardiac critical care are often shorter than in days gone by, whilst the technology moves on apace. A gap had arisen for a practical guide to the specialty written by experts suitable for use by trainees and more experienced clinicians in intensive care medicine, anaesthesia, and surgery alike. A strength of this volume is that it will not only be of use in specialist critical care, patients present to general intensive care units with significant cardiac and respiratory problems and this handbook contains many chapters relevant to all intensivists including up to date management of heart failure and cardiac pacing. Echo both transthoracic and transoesophageal, skills spilling out into wider critical care practice, are well covered.

A particular example of the utility of this book to the general intensivist and anaesthetist is the comprehensive chapter on the anatomical and physiological consequences of congenital heart disease, its treatment and long term sequelae. Clear descriptions and illustrations will help the non- specialist formulate care plans for the management of these complex patients when presenting for none cardiac surgery, obstetric care or as an emergency.

Oxford specialist handbooks are recognized as high quality, concise, and authoritarian, this volume is no exception. Writing and editing such a wide ranging and comprehensive textbook is an epic, indeed herculean task and the authors are to be commended for their efforts.

Anna Batchelor
Consultant in Anaesthesia and Intensive Care Medicine
Royal Victoria Infirmary
Newcastle, UK

Preface

This is an exciting time in intensive care medicine. The specialty has grown and matured rapidly from its early roots in anaesthesia. In the UK the formation of the new Faculty of Intensive Care Medicine marks an unequivocal coming of age. And yet, almost unnoticed, on the margins of the main story, another immensely significant development has been gathering pace; the crystallisation of *cardiothoracic* intensive care as a clinical entity in its own right. Just as general intensive care grew from the emergence of effective technologies to support the failing lung, so cardiothoracic intensive care has been catalysed by new and effective techniques of circulatory support.

Cardiothoracic intensive care has seen recent major developments in mechanical cardiovascular support (intra arterial balloon pump, ventricular assist devices and extracorporeal membrane oxygenation) and drug therapies such as nitric oxide and new inotropic agents. Clinical management has seen a dramatic shift from pragmatic, experience-based algorithms to care based on early diagnosis, proactive intervention and pathophysiological understanding. A major factor in this shift has been the development of sophisticated bed-side echocardiography.

The new clinical infant is still undeveloped. The shape of its future growth politically and clinically is not yet clear. Traditionally much of the workload has been based around care of patients after cardiac surgery, but new workstreams are developing rapidly, particularly in advanced heart failure and around cardiological interventions. One thing *is* clear, cardiothoracic intensive care is now at the cutting edge of intensive care medicine.

This book is primarily aimed at cardiothoracic intensive care residents, fellows and nursing staff. It is intended as a practical tool for those who find themselves in positions of responsibility, often at the start of a steep learning curve. It is a bedside handbook, not a textbook. It can be used as a quick clinical reference source, as a guide to deeper study and as an aide memoire. It provides an overview of the subspecialty focussing on the procedures, skills, guidelines, and technologies which are particular to *cardiothoracic* intensive care. It forms a complimentary text to companion volumes on cardiothoracic *anaesthesia* and *general* intensive care.

The material is grouped into four intuitive headings. These sections are broken up into brief chapters each focusing on a key topic and designed to allow quick access to relevant information. The style is deliberately didactic with boxes and bullet points, summary diagrams, key learning points and references for further reading. Where possible the material is based on evidence-based critical appraisal of recent trial studies and international guidelines and it follows British and European accreditation programmes.

The authors are all experienced practitioners in cardiothoracic critical care, but above all they are enthusiasts for their subject and the specialty. If this text supports the clinical development of a new generation of enthusiasts, it will have done its work well.

Contents

Symbols and Abbreviations

📖	cross-reference
↑	increased
↓	decreased
>	greater than
<	less than
⌧	website
~	approximately
2D	two-dimensional
ACE	angiotensin-converting enzyme
ACHD	adult congenital heart disease
ACR	albumin:creatinine ratio
ACS	acute coronary syndrome
ACT	activated clotting time
ACV	assist control ventilation
AF	atrial fibrillation
AHA	American Heart Association
AKI	acute kidney injury
ALI	acute lung injury
ALS	Advanced Life Support
APTT	activated partial thromboplastin time
AR	aortic regurgitation
ARDS	acute respiratory distress syndrome
AS	aortic stenosis
AUC	area under the curve
AV	atrioventricular
AVR	aortic valve replacement
BBB	bundle branch block
BIPAP	bi-level positive airway pressure
BMI	body mass index
BNP	brain natriuretic peptide
BP	blood pressure
BPF	bronchopleural fistula
CABG	coronary artery bypass graft
CALS	Cardiac Surgery Advanced Life Support
cAMP	cyclic adenosine monophosphate
CDI	*Clostridium difficile* infection

CF	cystic fibrosis
CFM	colour flow mapping
cGMP	cyclic guanosine monophosphate
CICU	cardiac intensive care unit
CKD	chronic kidney disease
CMV	cytomegalovirus
CNI	calcineurin inhibitor
CNS	central nervous system
CO	cardiac output
CO_2	carbon dioxide
COPD	chronic obstructive pulmonary disease
CPAP	continuous positive airway pressure
CPB	cardiopulmonary bypass
CPP	cerebral perfusion pressure
CPR	cardiopulmonary resuscitation
CRP	C-reactive protein
CRRT	continuous renal replacement therapy
CRT	cardiac resynchronization therapy
CT	computed tomography
CTx	cardiac transplantation
CVC	central venous cannulation
CVP	central venous pressure
CVS	cardiovascular system
CVVH	veno-venous haemofiltration
CWD	continuous wave Doppler
CXR	chest X-ray
DHCA	deep hypothermic circulatory arrest
DHF	decompensated heart failure
DLCO	carbon monoxide diffusing capacity
DLT	double-lumen tube
DVT	deep vein thrombosis
EACTS	European Association for Cardio-Thoracic Surgery
ECF	extracellular fluid
ECG	electrocardiogram
ECLS	extracorporeal lung support
ECMO	extracorporeal membrane oxygenation
EDD	end-diastolic dimension
EF	ejection fraction
eGFR	estimated glomerular filtration rate
ER	enhanced recovery

ERC	European Resuscitation Council
ESA	erythropoiesis stimulating agent
ESC	European Society of Cardiology
ESPEN	European Society for Parenteral and Enteral Nutrition
ETT	endotracheal tube
FATE	focus-assessed transthoracic echocardiography
FEV_1	forced expiratory volume in 1 second
FFP	fresh frozen plasma
GFR	glomerular filtration rate
GI	gastrointestinal
GTN	glyceryl trinitrate
HAI	hospital-acquired infection
hb	haemoglobin
HDU	high dependency unit
HIT	heparin induced thrombocytopenia
HOCM	hypertrophic obstructive cardiomyopathy
HR	heart rate
IABP	intra-aortic balloon pump
ICU	intensive care unit
IE	infective endocarditis
IJV	internal jugular vein
INR	international normalized ratio
IPAP	inspiratory positive airway pressure
IPF	idiopathic pulmonary fibrosis
IPPV	intermittent positive pressure ventilation
IRRT	intermittent renal replacement therapy
ITU	intensive therapy unit
IV	intravenous
JVP	jugular venous pressure
JVP	jugular venous pressure
K^+	potassium
KDIGO	Kidney Diseases: Improving Global Outcomes
L	litre
LAX	long axis
LBBB	left bundle branch block
LIMA	left internal mammary artery
LMWH	low-molecular-weight heparin
LTx	lung transplantation
LV	left ventricle/ventricular
LVAD	left ventricular assist device

LVEF	left ventricular ejection fraction
LVH	left ventricular hypertrophy
LVOT	left ventricular outflow tract
LVRS	lung volume reduction surgery
MAP	mean arterial pressure
mcg	microgram
MCS	mechanical circulatory support
mg	milligram
MI	myocardial infarction
MMF	mycophenolate mofetil
MR	mitral regurgitation
MRI	magnetic resonance imaging
MRSA	meticillin-resistant *Staphylococcus aureus*
MS	mitral stenosis
MV	mitral valve
MVO_2	myocardial oxygen consumption
MVP	mitral valve prolapse
NG	nasogastric
NIBP	non-invasive blood pressure
NICE	National Institute for Health and Clinical Excellence
NIV	non-invasive ventilation
NMDA	N-methyl-D-aspartate
NOMI	non-occlusive mesenteric ischaemia
NSAID	non-steroidal anti-inflammatory drug
NSR	normal sinus rhythm
NT-proBNP	N-terminal-pro brain natriuretic peptide
NYHA	New York Heart Association
O_2	oxygen
OOHCA	out-of-hospital cardiac arrest
PA	pulmonary artery
PAC	pulmonary artery catheter
PAFC	pulmonary artery flotation catheter
PAP	pulmonary artery pressure
PAWP	pulmonary artery wedge pressure
PCR	protein:creatinine ratio
PCWP	pulmonary capillary wedge pressure
PDA	posterior descending coronary artery
PE	pulmonary embolism
PEA	pulseless electrical activity
PEEP	positive end-expiratory pressure

PF	platelet factor
PFT	pulmonary function test
PISA	proximal isovelocity surface area
PPE	personal protective equipment
PPI	proton pump inhibitor
p-SIMV	pressure synchronized intermittent mandatory ventilation
PSV	pressure support ventilation
PT	prothrombin time
PVR	pulmonary vascular resistance
PW	pressure wave
PWD	pulsed wave Doppler
RCA	right coronary artery
ROSC	return of spontaneous circulation
RRT	renal replacement therapy
RV	right ventricle/ventricular
RVAD	right ventricular assist device
SAM	systolic anterior motion
SAX	short axis
SBE	standard base excess
SCV	subclavian vein
SIMV	synchronized intermittent mandatory ventilation
SIRS	systemic inflammatory response syndrome
SMR	standardized mortality ratio
SpO_2	saturation of peripheral oxygen
SV	stroke volume
SVC	superior vena cava
SvO_2	mixed venous oxygen saturation
SVR	systemic vascular resistance
TCI	target-controlled infusion
TOE	transoesophageal echocardiography
TPN	total parenteral nutrition
TR	tricuspid regurgitation
TS	tricuspid stenosis
TTE	transthoracic echocardiography
TV	tricuspid valve
V/Q	ventilation/perfusion
VAC	vacuum-assisted closure
VAD	ventricular assist device
VAP	ventilator-associated pneumonia
VAS	Visual Analogue Scale

VATS	video-assisted thoracoscopic surgery
VCV	volume controlled ventilation
VF	ventricular fibrillation
VILI	ventilator-induced lung injury
VSD	ventricular septal defect
VT	ventricular tachycardia
VTE	venous thromboembolism
VTI	velocity-time integral

Contributors

Lynne Anderson
Consultant Anaesthetitst
Department of Anaesthesia
Golden Jubilee National Hospital
Clydebank, UK

Michael Brett
Anaesthetics and Intensive Care
Medicine
Royal Alexandra Hospital
Paisley, UK

Anton Buter
Consultant General Surgeon
General Surgery
Royal Alexandra Hospital
Paisley, UK

Coralie Carle
Consultant in Anaesthesia and
Critical Care Medicine
Peterborough City Hospital
Peterborough,UK

Ian Colquhoun
Consultant Cardiothoracic Surgeon
West of Scotland Heart and
Lung Unit
Golden Jubilee National Hospital
Clydebank, UK

Mark Davidson
Paediatric Intensivist
Paediatric Intensive Care Unit
Royal Hospital for Sick Children
Glasgow, UK

Joel Dunning
Cardiothoracic Unit
James Cook University Hospital
Middlesbrough, UK

Clare Gardner
Consultant Anaesthetist
St John's Hospital
Livingston, UK

Roy Gardner
Scottish National Advanced Heart
Failure Service
Golden Jubilee National Hospital
Clydebank, UK

Donna Greenhalgh
Consultant in Cardiothoracic
Anaesthesia
University Hospital of South
Manchester
Stockport UK

Doshi Harikrishna
Department of Congenital Cardiac
Surgery
Alder Hey Children's Hospital
Liverpool, UK

Chris Hawthorne
Clinical Lecturer
Academic Unit of Anaesthesia,
Pain and Critical Care Medicine
University of Glasgow
Glasgow, UK

Stephen Hickey
Department of Anaesthesia
Golden Jubilee National Hospital
Clydebank, UK

Mike Higgins
Medical Director
Golden Jubilee National Hospital
Clydebank, UK

Martin Hughes
Consultant in Anaesthesia and
Intensive Care Medicine
Intensive Care Unit
Glasgow Royal Infirmary
Glasgow, UK

Theresa Inkster
Consultant Microbiologist
Department of Microbiology
Glasgow Royal Infirmary
Glasgow, UK

Nitish Khanna
Consultant Microbiologist
Department of Microbiology
Southern General Hospital
Glasgow, UK

Adarsh Lal
Department of Anaesthesia
Golden Jubilee National Hospital
Clydebank, UK

Ninian Lang
Clinical Lecturer in Cardiology
University of Edinburgh
Edinburgh, UK

Alistair Macfie
Department of Anaesthesia
Golden Jubilee National Hospital
Clydebank, UK

Ken McKinlay
Consultant in Anaesthesia and
Intensive Care
Department of Anaesthesia
Golden Jubilee National Hospital
Clydebank, UK

Naomi May
Specialist Registrar in Anaesthetics
Department of Anaesthetics
West of Scotland
Glasgow, UK

Neal Padmanabhan
Consultant Nephrologist
Renal Unit
Western Infirmary
Glasgow, UK

John Payne
Scottish National Advanced Heart
Failure Service
Golden Jubilee National Hospital
Clydebank, UK

Jorg Prinzlin
Department of Anaesthesia
Golden Jubilee National Hospital
Clydebank, UK

Isma Quasim
Department of Anaesthesia
Golden Jubilee National Hospital
Clydebank, UK

Stefan Schraag
Department of Anaesthesia
Golden Jubilee National Hospital
Clydebank, UK

Jason Shahin
Department of Critical Care
Division of pulmonary medicine
McGill University
Montreal, Quebec, Canada

Ben Shelley
Clinical Research Fellow
University of Glasgow
Glasgow, UK

Andrew Sinclair
Department of Anaesthesia
Golden Jubilee National Hospital
Clydebank, UK

Robyn Smith
Department of Anaesthesia
Golden Jubilee National Hospital
Clydebank, UK

Tim Strang
Department of Anaesthesia
University of South Manchester
Manchester, UK

Alison Taylor
Registrar in Nephrology
Glasgow Renal and Transplant Unit
Western Infirmary
Glasgow, UK

Niki Walker
Consultant Cardiologist
Golden Jubilee National Hospital
Clydebank, UK

Stephen Webb
Department of Anaesthesia and
Intensive Care
Papworth Hospital NHS
Foundation Trust
Cambridge, UK

Alice Young
Dietitian
Golden Jubilee National Hospital
Clydebank, UK

Early postoperative management

Chapter 1

The normal postoperative cardiac patient

Introduction

Cardiac surgery involves considerable physiological trespass. Nevertheless, most cardiac patients recover uneventfully with comfortable margins of safety.

However, a small proportion of routine patients develop an important treatable complication. A second small group of patients are critically ill and are dependant on exact optimization of their physiology, either because of their preoperative condition or their operative course or both. The latter group are usually obvious and are often already on substantial support and invasive monitoring when they leave theatre. Recognizing the first group is crucial and is a key skill of cardiac intensive care. The key to success with these patients is early proactive management. In turn, this requires attention to detail, an understanding of normal postoperative course, close serial observation, and excellent diagnosis employing early use of additional monitoring and investigation.

Effects of surgery and cardiopulmonary bypass

Inflammatory response

Major surgery and cardiopulmonary bypass (CPB) both cause a systemic inflammatory response. All patients who have undergone cardiac surgery will have some degree of inflammatory activation, even those who have undergone off-pump surgery. In a substantial proportion of patients this response will be clinically apparent and in a small fraction it will be problematic.

Cooling

During CPB patients are often cooled to 32°C or lower. Despite initial re-warming, after separation from bypass there may be a re-distribution of heat to poorly perfused tissues leading to an 'after drop' in core temperature. Once anaesthesia wears off, the low core temperature will trigger reflex shivering. This in turn leads to ↑ cardiac output (CO) and ↑ respiratory workload to service the muscle activity. Re-warming normally occurs at 0.5–2°C/hour and is dependent on a normal CO and blood volume.

Pulmonary effects

Gas exchange is often measurably impaired after cardiac surgery. This is due to a combination of causes including atelectasis as a result of anaesthesia and lung collapse during CPB, and ↑ lung water secondary to the inflammatory response. Relatively large doses of opioid drugs may be used during cardiac anaesthesia which may result in postoperative respiratory depression. Conversely, pain contributes to atelectasis and impaired gas exchange.

Urine output and fluid balance

Patients have significant fluid derangements as a result of CPB. There is a fluid load as a result of the pump-prime which leads to an increase in total body fluid. However, the intravascular space may be depleted as a result of capillary leak. The kidneys are at risk of insult from CPB. There is a tradition of giving the osmotic diuretic mannitol during bypass to promote clearance of excess fluid. This leads to high postoperative urine volumes in the first few hours after surgery. However, at the same time patients commonly require a positive fluid balance to maintain pre-load because of inflammatory activation.

Pain

Pain immediately after median sternotomy is generally less problematic than after major abdominal surgery and can be managed by a range of appropriate techniques.

Cardiac function

Cardiac contractility may be adversely affected by ischaemia during bypass or intraoperative handling and by reperfusion injury (stunning). This process may worsen in the first few hours after surgery.

Bleeding

CPB is associated with abnormal haemostasis through a series of mechanisms involving coagulopathy, ↑ fibrinolysis, haemodilution, and qualitative and quantitative platelet dysfunction. Only a minority of patients will have a clinically significant lesion.

Typical progression

The following represents patients following a traditional progression. This may be modified by modern enhanced recovery techniques.

On admission
- Cold core (34–36°C)
- Large core–peripheral gradient (10°C)
- Polyuric
- Deeply sedated
- Fully ventilated
- Good gas exchange
- Variable mediastinal drainage
- Normal coagulation
- Variable inotrope and pressor support
- Anaemic (haemoglobin (Hb) 70–110g/L)
- Supine position
- High/normal blood glucose
- May be relatively bradycardic and pacing dependent.

First hour
- Increasing core temp (0.5–2°C over the hour)
- Core–peripheral gradient remains high
- May shiver
- High urine output (100–300mL/h)
- Remains sedated
- Gas exchange stable
- Drain loss up to 200mL
- Variable pressor support but often tendency to hypotension requiring moderate volume transfusion 500–1000mL (± low-dose pressors)
- May have increasing or decreasing inotrope requirements
- May require insulin to control blood glucose
- Falling K$^+$ requires supplementation.

1–4 hours
- Rewarmed to 36.8°
- Core–peripheral gradient normalized (<3°C)
- Urine output tapering to normal (0.5–1mL/kg/hour)
- Sat up >30°: gas exchange stable or improving with posture change
- Stabilized blood pressure (BP) with
- Stabilized pressor requirements
- Stabilized low inotrope requirement
- Decreasing volume requirements
- Stable and normal acid–base levels
- Commonly in positive fluid balance (up to 1L)
- Decreasing mediastinal drainage tapering to <50mL/hour
- Usually stable/increasing haematocrit (capillary leak); Hb >70g/L
- Gas exchange good or improving
- Normal or slightly raised (>7.0) CO_2 (mild narcotization)
- Minimal sedation and interacting purposefully

- Low/no pain
- Breathing spontaneously
- Interacting purposefully
- May be extubated
- May require insulin to control blood glucose
- Falling K$^+$ requires supplementation
- Stabilizing rhythm (decreasing pacing dependence).

4–6 hours

- As for 1–4 hours
- Often ↓ pressor requirements as sedation stopped
- Most are extubated.

Routine management

The majority of patients require minimal intervention and are best served by following routine protocols.

Ventilation

Patients are usually ventilated for several hours after cardiac surgery. Typical ventilator settings employ relatively low tidal volumes (0.7mL/kg) with a small amount of positive end-expiratory pressure (PEEP) (5cmH$_2$O) to counteract atelectasis. Patients are weaned onto a spontaneous breathing mode as soon as possible. Patients should be extubated once they reach the required criteria and do not need progressive weaning of mechanical support. A relatively high CO$_2$ is likely to indicate narcosis rather than respiratory muscle insufficiency and may be tolerated if otherwise clinically appropriate.

Extubation criteria
- Awake and responding to requests
- Comfortable
- Sustained spontaneous respirations
- FiO$_2$ <0.5 with SaO$_2$ >95%
- CO$_2$ <7.0kPa
- Core temperature ≥36.8°C
- No excessive blood loss (see 📖 Fluid and electrolyte management, p. 9)
- Cardiovascularly stable.

Re-warming
- Re-warming may be passive or aided by warm-air re-warmers.
- Shivering should be suppressed by increasing sedation, treating with pethidine 25–50mg IV, or, if severe, by non-depolarizing muscle relaxants (in this case patient must be unconscious).

Inotropes and vasopressors

Routine patients may require *low doses* (e.g. up to 0.1mcg/kg/min of adrenaline or noradrenaline or 8mcg/kg/min of dopamine) of inotropes or vasopressors in the first few hours after operation. In general, noradrenalin as a sole agent should be reserved to use in patients with good ventricular function. Inotropes and pressors can often be weaned over the first few hours after operation. Physiological targets vary from patient to patient (see 📖 Postoperative hypotension, p. 49). Relative hypotension can be tolerated if there is good evidence of adequate perfusion (e.g. normal urine output, normal cerebration, good peripheral perfusion).

Fluid and electrolyte management
- Maintain K$^+$ 4.5–6.0mmol/L
- Insulin to keep glucose management is 5.0–10.0mmol/L (see 📖 Glucose, p. 65)
- Colloids as required to maintain pre-load
- Oral fluids once extubated.
- Transfuse packed red cells to keep Hb >70g/dL.

Analgesia and antiemesis

There is no single agreed optimum postoperative analgesic regimen. An acceptable approach includes the following elements:

- Opioids titrated to effect
- Antiemetics (e.g. ondansetron 10mg IV, buccal prochlorperazine 3mg) as required
- Regular paracetamol 1g 6-hourly.

Warning signs

Any of the following should prompt clinical review and careful ongoing attention:

- Failure to warm
- Increasing base excess (worse than −5)
- High or increasing lactate (>3.0mmol/L)
- Hypotension unresponsive to fluid challenge or low-dose vasopressor (0.1mcg/kg noradrenaline)
- Oliguria (<0.5mL/kg/min or <1mL/kg/min in the first 3 hours if the patient has had mannitol)
- Poor peripheral perfusion
- Low cardiac index (<2.2L/m^2)
- Excessive chest drainage:
  - >300mL in first hour
  - >200mL each hour for any 2 consecutive hours
  - >150mL each hour for any 4 consecutive hours
- High central venous pressure (CVP) (>15mmHg)
- FiO$_2$ >0.5 to maintain normal saturation
- Frequent or sustained dysrhythmia
- >2L positive fluid balance over first 12 hours.

Risk prediction and outcome

Prognostic models

Prognostic models allow the prediction of patient outcomes in intensive care units (ICUs) based on multiple risk factors. They are often referred to as prognostic models, risk prediction models, or severity of illness scores.

What are prognostic models?

- Statistical models using commonly measured risk factors to predict patient outcome.
- Risk factors usually consist of:
  - Physiological variables
  - Chronic health conditions
  - ICU admission diagnosis.
- Usually measured within first 24 hours of ICU admission.
- Hospital mortality is the most common and reliable outcome.

Commonly used prognostic models for adult general ICUs include:
- APACHE (Acute Physiology and Chronic Health Evaluation—Table 2.1)
- SAPS (Simplified Acute Physiology Score)
- MPM (Mortality Probability Model)
- ICNARC (Intensive Care National Audit & Research Centre).

How are prognostic models developed?

- Accurate data on risk factors and outcomes are collected prospectively.
- Risk factors are chosen based on literature review, existing prognostic models, and expert opinion.
- Model is developed using regression techniques.
- Relative weights are assigned to risk factors based on regression model.
- Model performance is assessed by testing for discrimination (ability to discriminate between individuals with and without the outcome) and calibration (how well the model mirrors the true outcome rate).

What are prognostic models used for?

By controlling for differences in risk, prognostic models allow clinicians, managers, policymakers, patients, and relatives to make informed decisions. The most common examples are:
- *Benchmarking*: to assess quality of care delivered by ICUs using standardized mortality ratios (SMRs):
  - SMR is the ratio of observed deaths to expected deaths (estimated by the model) and is used to compare an ICU to a reference group (e.g. the national average).
- *Performance assessment*: to allow ICUs to compare current performance with past performance.
- *Resource utilization*: to allow appropriate resource allocation to ICUs.
- *Clinical trials*: to select patients for inclusion into clinical trials based on risk.
- *Clinical decision-making*: as a bedside clinical decision-making tool:
  - Has not been validated for this use and may not be accurate.

Table 2.1 APACHE II score

Acute Physiology score	Score								
	4	3	2	1	0	1	2	3	4
Temperature (°C)	≤29.9	30–31.9	32–33.9	34–35.9	36–38.4	38.5–38.9		39–40.9	≥41
Mean arterial pressure (mmHg)	≤49		50–69		70–109		110–129	130–159	≥160
Heart rate	≤39	40–54	55–69		70–109		110–139	140–179	≥180
Respiratory rate (non-ventilated or ventilated)	≤5		6–9	10–11	12–24	25–34		35–49	≥50
Oxygenation status									
A–a gradient mmHg (if FiO$_2$ ≥0.5)					<200		200–349	350–499	≥500
PaO$_2$ mmHg (if FiO$_2$ <0.5)	<55	55–60	61–70		>70				
Acid–base status									
Arterial pH (if ABG present)	≥7.7	7.6–7.69		7.5–7.59	7.33–7.49		7.25–7.32	7.15–7.24	<7.15
Serum HCO$_3$ (mEq/L) (if no ABG)	≥52	41–51.9	32–40.9		22–31.9		18–21.9	15–17.9	<15
Serum NA (mmol/L)	≥180	160–179	155–159	150–154	130–149		120–129	111–119	≤110
Serum K (mmol/L)	≥7	6–6.9		5.5–5.9	3.5–5.4		3–3.4	2.5–2.9	<2.5
Serum creatinine (μmol/L) no acute renal failure[a]	≥305	170–304	130–169		54–129				<54

(Continued)

Table 2.1 (Continued)

Acute Physiology score	Score							
	4	3	2	1	0	1	2	3	4
Hematocrit (%)	≥60		50–59.9	46–49.9	30–45.9		20–29.9		<20
White blood cell count (× 10³/mm³)	≥40		20–39.9	15–19.9	3–14.9		1–2.9		<1

GCS: score is 15 – actual GCS

Total Acute Physiology score= sum of above points.

Total APACHE score = Acute physiology score + age points + chronic health points.

Diagnostic category weight: final score is modified depending on diagnosis.

*Double points if acute renal failure.

ABG: arterial blood gas; GCS: Glasgow Coma Score.

Data from Knaus et al., 'APACHE II: A severity of disease classification system', *Critical Care Medicine*, 13, 10, pp. 818–829, 1985, The Williams & Wilkins Co.

Organ failure scores

Unlike prognostic models, organ failure models assess the degree of organ dysfunction in major organ systems (cardiovascular, respiratory, renal, hepatic, haematological, neurological):
- Can be measured daily (not restricted to first 24 hours of admission)
- Points allocated based on degree of organ dysfunction
- Easy to calculate
- Allows ICU monitoring of ICU trajectory
- Not initially designed for risk prediction
- Gastrointestinal (GI) and endocrine systems are not included because of difficulty in assessment of degree of organ dysfunction.

Commonly used organ failure models for adult general ICUs include:
- SOFA (Sequential Organ Failure Assessment)
- MODS (Multiple Organ Dysfunction Score)
- LODS (Logistic Organ Dysfunction System).

Cardiac surgery prognostic models

Death after cardiac surgery is related to the patient's preoperative risk profile. Hospital mortality is used as a marker of quality of care after cardiac
surgery. In order to compare hospital mortality rates for different hospitals
and different surgeons, patients' preoperative risk profiles must be adjusted
using the patient preoperative risk profile.

Commonly used preoperative cardiac surgery prognostic models include:
- EuroSCORE
- Parsonnet Score.

EuroSCORE

- Developed using a cohort of 14,799 patients from 128 hospitals in eight
  European countries.
- Widely used across Europe.
- The model consists of three groups of risk factors:
  - Patient-related factors
  - Cardiac-related factors
  - Operation-related factors.
- Two models exist (Table 2.2).
- Additive model:
  - Simple to use
  - Can be calculated at bedside
  - Simple addition of points
  - Underestimates risk in high-risk groups.
- Logistic model:
  - Uses logistic equation
  - Same risk factors as additive model
  - Better suited for high-risk patients.
- A revised score is being developed—*EuroSCORE 2010*:
  - Being developed in >300 centres in different countries
  - Expected to provide more accurate risk prediction for a diverse
    patient population
  - EuroSCORE calculator can be found at ℰ <http://euroscore.org/
    index.htm>.

Parsonnet score

- Redeveloped in 2000 using a cohort of 10,703 patients in 10 US centres.
- Calculation is based on simple addition of scores with graphical
  interpretation (Fig. 2.1).
- Helpful as a guide to patients and family in estimating cardiac
  surgical risk.

Table 2.2 EuroSCORE additive and logistic regression models

Risk factor	Description	Points	β coefficient
Patient-related factors			
Age	Per 5 years or part thereof >60 years	1	0.0666354
Sex	Female	1	0.3304052
Serum creatinine	>200 µmol/L	2	0.6521653
Extracardiac arteriopathy	Any 1 or more of the following: claudication, carotid occlusion or >50% stenosis, previous or planned intervention on the abdominal aorta, limb arteries, or carotids	2	0.6558917
Pulmonary disease	Long-term use of bronchodilators or steroids for lung disease	1	0.4931341
Neurological dysfunction	Disease severely affecting ambulation or day-to-day functioning	2	0.841626
Critical preoperative status	Any 1 or more of the following: ventricular tachycardia or fibrillation or aborted sudden death, preoperative cardiac massage, preoperative ventilation before arrival in the anaesthetic room, preoperative inotropic support, intra-aortic balloon counterpulsation or preoperative acute renal failure (anuria or oliguria <10mL/h)	3	0.9058132
Active endocarditis	Patient still under antibiotic treatment for endocarditis at the time of surgery	3	1.101265
Previous cardiac surgery	Requiring opening of the pericardium	3	1.002625
Cardiac-related factors			
Unstable angina	Rest angina requiring IV nitrates until arrival in the anaesthetic room	2	0.5677075
Recent MI	<90 days	2	0.5460218
LV dysfunction	LVEF 30–50%	1	0.4191643
	LVEF <30%	3	1.094443
Pulmonary hypertension	Systolic PAP >60mmHg	2	0.7676924

(Continued)

Table 2.2 (Continued)

Risk factor	Description	Points	β coefficient
Operation-related factors			
Emergency operation	Carried out on referral before the beginning of the next working day	2	0.7127953
Ventricular septal rupture		4	1.462009
Other than isolated coronary surgery	Major cardiac procedure other than or in addition to CABG	2	0.5420364
Thoracic aortic surgery	For disorder of ascending arch or descending aorta	3	1.159787

CABG: coronary artery bypass graft; IV: intravenous; LV: left ventricular; LVEF: left ventricular ejection fraction; MI: myocardial infarction; PAP: pulmonary artery pressure.
Data from Roques F, Michel P, Goldstone AR, Nashef SAM, 'The logistic EuroSCORE', *European Heart Journal*, 2003, 24, 9, pp. 1–2, Oxford University Press and European Society of Cardiology.

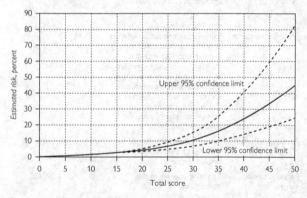

Figure 2.1 Graphic tool used to calculate risk score. Reprinted from *The Annals of Thoracic Society*, 69, 3, AD Bernstein and V Parsonnet, 'Bedside estimation of risk as an aid for decision-making in cardiac surgery', pp. 823–828, Copyright 2000, with permission from Elsevier and the American Thoracic Society.

Further reading

Afessa B, Gajic O, Keegan MT. Severity of illness and organ failure assessment in adult intensive care units. *Crit Care Clinics* 2007;23:639–58.

Altman DG, Vergouwe Y, Royston P, Moons KGM. Prognosis and prognostic research: validating a prognostic model. *BMJ* 2009;338:605.

Bernstein AD, Parsonnet V. Bedside estimation of risk as an aid for decision making in cardiac surgery. *Ann Thorac Surg* 2000;69:823–8.

Nashef SAM, Roques F, Michel P, Gauducheau E, Lemeshow S, Salamon R. European system for cardiac operative risk evaluation (EuroSCORE). *Eur J Cardiothorac Surg* 1999;16:9–13.

Roques F, Michel P, Goldstone AR, Nashef SAM. The logistic EuroSCORE. *Eur Heart J* 2003;24:1–2.

Chapter 3

Fast-tracking the low-risk patient

Fast-track concepts

Achieving a rapid and sustained recovery is one of the primary goals in the modern management of cardiac surgical patients.

Advancements in surgery, anaesthesia, and improved patient selection and preparation have led to the development of fast-track programmes.

The defining characteristic of these programmes is the reduction in the use of critical care resources in the postoperative period. Instead, the patient is managed in a specialized recovery of postsurgical care unit and stepped down to the cardiac surgical ward directly from there.

Principles of fast-tracking the low-risk patient

The key elements are:

- *Patient*: low risk profile, preserved ventricular function, minimal co-morbidity.
- *Surgery*: attention to good haemostasis, minimal blood loss, and meticulous wound management
- *Anaesthesia*: achieving haemodynamic stability and using short-acting anaesthetic drugs.
- *Recovery unit*: aggressive normothermia, no postoperative sedation, clear bleeding protocol, tight extubation protocol.

Applying these principles has been shown to be equally safe for the patient when compared to the traditional critical care pathway.

When looking at the overall in-hospital mortality in a series of almost 8000 patients, a retrospective analysis could not demonstrate an increased risk of adverse outcome when compared to historical controls.

However, this publication also showed that in spite achieving faster initial recovery and extubation, this not necessarily translated in shorter hospital length of stay and stresses the need that working fast-track concepts should be part of a wider enhanced recovery (ER) programme to utilize its potential.

Examples of fast-track protocols

Two major versions of fast-track protocols after cardiac surgery have been described. They share similarities, but depend on the hospital's resources and infrastructure.

- *The recovery room concept* (Fig. 3.1): this means that the patient is either extubated in theatre and then transferred to the theatre's main recovery room or extubation will take place there shortly after arrival. The patient is looked after by specially trained recovery nurses and a dedicated anaesthetist and surgeon overlook the patient's recovery, able to troubleshoot if required. When achieving predefined criteria, the patient is discharged straight to the surgical high dependency unit (HDU).
- *The cardiac recovery unit concept* (Fig. 3.2): in this version the hospital provides a special unit of recovery beds close to theatres. All suitable patients will be admitted either extubated or they will be recovered according to strict protocols that are designed to avoid unnecessary delays. Once a patient has achieved a certain level of recovery they will be discharged to HDU. Dependent on the capacity, there is the

option to recover the patient further without moving them for another 24 hours, followed by a discharge straight to the ward.

Both models include the option that any patient who deteriorates or for other reasons is not suitable for either concept will be admitted in the ICU.

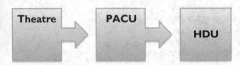

Figure 3.1   The recovery room concept. Reproduced from Dunning J et al., 'Guideline for resuscitation in cardiac arrest after cardiac surgery', *European Journal of Cardio-Thoracic Surgery*, 2009, 36, pp. 3–28, by permission of the European Association for Cardio-Thoracic Surgery, the European Society of Thoracic Surgeons, and Oxford University Press.

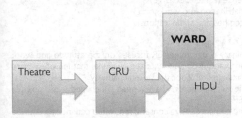

Figure 3.2   The cardiac recovery unit concept. Reproduced from Dunning J et al., 'Guideline for resuscitation in cardiac arrest after cardiac surgery', *European Journal of Cardio-Thoracic Surgery*, 2009, 36, pp. 3–28, by permission of the European Association for Cardio-Thoracic Surgery, the European Society of Thoracic Surgeons, and Oxford University Press.

Further reading

Ender J, Borger MA, Scholz M, Funkat AK, Anwar N, Sommer M, et al. Cardiac surgery fast-track treatment in a postanesthetic care unit. *Anesthesiology* 2008;109:61–6.

Häntschel D, Fassl J, Scholz M, Sommer M, Funkat AK, Wittmann M, et al. Leipzig "Fast-track" protocol in cardiac anaesthesia. Effective, safe and economical. *Anaesthesist* 2009;58:379–86.

Svircevic V, Nierich AP, Moons KG, Brandon Bravo Bruinsma GJ, Kalkman CJ, van Dijk D. Fast-track anesthesia and cardiac surgery: A retrospective cohort study of 7989 patients. *Anesth Analg* 2009;108:727–33.

Enhanced recovery

What is enhanced recovery?

ER is a high-quality surgical care pathway and a concept to get patients better, sooner. The major goals behind ER are:

- To reduce morbidity and mortality
- To allow stable mental recovery
- To reduce hospital length of stay
- To improve functional capacity
- To reduce inflammatory response
- To reduce development of chronic pain.

This development was influenced and supported by improved and less invasive surgical techniques, better understanding of controlling surgical pain, newer and cleaner general and local anaesthetics, and more evidence-based perioperative supportive care.

The potential improvements with ER for cardiac surgical patients include:

- Savings (ICU, staff, improved capacity)
- Patient experience (earlier discharge)
- Economic (rehabilitation into work force)
- Clinical (reduced hospital complications).

Components of ER

As a multidisciplinary programme, ER focuses on the attitude and work ethic of combining various components and elements that individually are evidence-based and applicable for the surgical pathway.

The following components have been identified as positive contributors to ER:

- Pre-assessment: comprehensive consent, motivated patient
- Scheduling: suitable surgical teams and resources
- Patient preparation: reduce fasting times, allow carbohydrate drinks
- Surgical technique: minimal invasive procedures, haemostasis, normothermia, local anaesthesia
- Anaesthetic technique: short-acting drugs, regional anaesthesia, cardiovascular stability
- Early extubation
- Drains: timely removal of chest drains, central venous lines and urinary catheter
- Physiotherapy: intense chest physiotherapy and mobilization
- Nutrition: early oral nutrition and balanced diet.

Further reading

Holte K, Kehlet H. Fluid therapy and surgical outcomes in elective surgery: a need for reassessment in fast-track surgery. *J Am Coll Surg* 2006;202:971–89.

Kehlet H. Fast-track surgery. An update on physiological care principles to enhance recovery. *Langenbecks Arch Surg* 2011;396:585–90.

Wilmore DW, Kehlet H. Management of patients in fast-track surgery. *BMJ* 2001;322:473–6.

Resuscitation in the cardiac intensive care setting

Cardiac Surgery Advanced Life Support

The Cardiac Surgery Advanced Life Support (CALS) course was developed in response to recognized differences which are required for management of arrested patients post sternotomy in contrast to standard European Resuscitation Council (ERC) Advanced Life Support (ALS) guidelines. CALS forms the European Association for Cardio-Thoracic Surgery (EACTS) guidelines.

These modifications to standard ALS have now been taken on by the ERC and incorporated into the 'Special Situation – post cardiac surgery' section. The following text therefore relates only to patients up to 10 days post sternotomy who arrest on a cardiac ICU (CICU).

Differences from 'standard' ward arrest

- Many more available skilled staff members.
- Arrest is identified immediately.
- Much wider range of possible therapies.
- Patient is often highly monitored and intubated.
- Chest re-opening is a standard part of resuscitation—indeed when considering the 4Hs and 4Ts in the post-sternotomy setting all are resolved by chest opening as the cause of arrest on the CICU is often mechanical, e.g. tamponade, blown graft, loss of pacing.

Key components of arrest management

- Early identification of patient pre-arrest.
- Key specific roles for team members on arrival at scene.
- Adoption of modified protocol regarding defibrillation/drugs (see Fig. 4.1).
- Use of simplified chest opening kit.
- Use of 'all in one' sterile drape (central adhesive window)—no prep to wound.
- Successful outcome in 48% if chest opened rapidly.

Key specific roles and modifications from 'standard' ALS

See Fig. 4.2.

Identification of arrest

- Do not be sidetracked by monitor traces!
- Defibrillate or pace before massage if equipment at bedside.
- Efficacy of massage can be judged from A line trace.
- Switch intra-aortic balloon pump (IABP) to pressure mode.

Airway role

- Identification of tension pneumothorax may be difficult in a noisy ICU environment.

Defibrillation

- In ventricular fibrillation (VF) three shocks are administered before chest opening—anticipate the need for internal paddles.
- Asystole—attach pacer, DDD, rate 90, maximum output, anticipate the need for internal wires.
- Pulseless electrical activity (PEA)—turn off pacer to unmask covert VF.

Team leader

- Make early decision to open chest.
- Gown and glove, rapidly minimal (if any) hand wash.
- Do not apply cleaning agents to wound—these work by drying and delay opening.
- Apply 'all-in-one drape' to patient after massager has removed wound dressing.
- Massage over sterile dressing until chest opening kit delivered.
- Open chest, deliver internal massage/shocks, identify cause of arrest.

Drugs

- Do *NOT* give adrenaline (will cause catastrophic hypertension once tamponade relieved). Stop all infusions especially if drug error a possibility.

Coordinator role

- Coordinate sending for help.
- Assist others to rapidly gown and deliver opening kit.

Pitfalls of chest opening

- Note scalpel cannot be packaged in a sterile kit—use disposable scalpel.
- Chest opening itself is harmless—even without sternal retraction tamponade may be resolved.
- Internal massage can carry hazards—avoid dislodging left internal mammary artery (LIMA), grafts, and pacing wires.
- Only use two-handed technique—one placed gently posterior to LV.
- Single-handed technique may result in thumb through right ventricle (RV) or annular disruption!

Contents of emergency reopening pack (only 5 items)

- Sternal retractors
- Wire cutters
- Large forceps
- Scissors
- Heavy needle holder.

Further reading

Dunning J, Fabbri A, Kolh PH, Levine A, Lockowandt U, Mackay J, et al. Guideline for resuscitation in cardiac arrest after cardiac surgery. *Eur J Cardiothorac Surg* 2009;36:3–28. ℘ <http://ejcts.oxfordjournals.org/content/36/1/3.long>.

Dunning J, Nandi J, Ariffin S, Jerstice J, Danitsch D, Levine A. The Cardiac Surgery Advanced Life Support Course (CALS): delivering significant improvements in emergency cardiothoracic care, *Ann Thorac Surg* 2006;81(5):1767–72. ℘ <http://dx.doi.org/10.1016/j.athoracsur.2005.12.012>.

Mackay JH, Powell SJ, Osgathorp J, Rozario CJ. Six-year prospective audit of chest reopening after cardiac arrest. *Eur J Cardiothorac Surg* 2002;22(3):421–5.

The Cardiac Surgery Advanced Life Support course: ℘ <http://www.csu-als.com>.

A video of this protocol in practice can be found at: ℘ http://www.youtube.com/watch?v=PHgYZDgQJgc

A handbook of this protocol can be found at: ℘ <http://www.lulu.com/content/4428266>.

CALS manual: ℘ <http://webapp.doctors.org.uk/Redirect/www.lulu.com/content/442826>.

Demonstration of chest opening: ℘ <http://webapp.doctors.org.uk/Redirect/www.youtube.com/watch?v=PHgYZDgQJgc>.

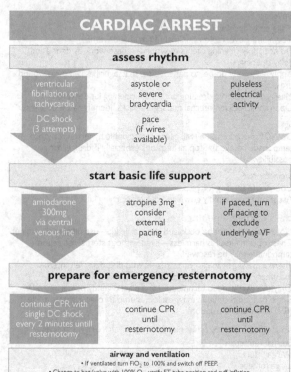

Figure 4.1 Arrest protocol. Reproduced from Dunning J. et al., 'Guideline for resuscitation in cardiac arrest after cardiac surgery', *European Journal of Cardio-thoracic Surgery*, 2009, 36, pp. 3–28, by permission of the European Association for Cardio-Thoracic Surgery, the European Society of Thoracic Surgeons, and Oxford University Press.

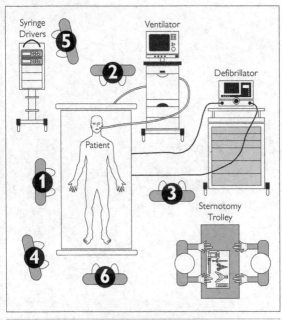

Six key roles in the cardiac arrest:
1. External cardiac massage
2. Airway and breathing
3. Defibrillation
4. Team leader
5. Drugs and syringe drivers
6. ICU co-ordinator

Figure 4.2 Six key roles in a cardiac arrest. Reproduced from Dunning J. et al., 'Guideline for resuscitation in cardiac arrest after cardiac surgery', *European Journal of Cardio-thoracic Surgery*, 2009, 36, pp. 3–28, by permission of the European Association for Cardio-Thoracic Surgery, the European Society of Thoracic Surgeons, and Oxford University Press.

Chapter 5

Myocardial ischaemia and infarction

Introduction

Myocardial ischaemia is an important cause of myocardial dysfunction in cardiac surgical patients in the postoperative period.

It is essential that the signs of myocardial ischaemia are recognized and treated early before a vicious deteriorating spiral culminating in MI occurs. The possible causes of myocardial ischaemia are:

- An imbalance of supply/demand balance resulting in subendocardial ischaemia
- Spasm of coronary artery or arterial conduit
- Thrombosis and/or occlusion of coronary graft or native coronary artery
- Mechanical issues such as kinking of a coronary artery graft related to CABG surgery.

How to diagnose myocardial ischaemia

In the CICU, clinical situations to consider myocardial ischaemia include:
- Unanticipated myocardial failure
- ST changes in pattern consistent with a distribution of coronary artery of graft
- ST elevation or depression which is episodic which may suggest coronary spasm
- Echocardiogram may show a new wall-motion abnormality
- Angina type pain may be present in the awake patient.

The right coronary artery (RCA) supplies the inferior and inferoseptal walls of the LV and much of the RV (Fig. 5.1). Electrocardiogram (ECG) changes will be seen in the inferior standard leads II, III, and aVF.

The left anterior descending branch of the left coronary artery supplies the anterior and anteroseptal walls. ECG changes will be seen in standard lead 1 and anterior chest leads V1–3.

The circumflex artery branch of the left coronary artery supplies the lateral and posterior wall of the LV. ECG changes will be seen in standard lead 1 and lateral ventricular lead aVL.

In 85% of patients the RCA is said to be 'dominant' because it supplies circulation to the inferior portion of the interventricular septum via the right posterior descending coronary artery (or PDA) branch.

Non-specific ST and T wave changes are common after cardiac surgery and may be due to pericardial reaction which makes recognition of myocardial ischaemic difficult. Intraventricular conduction defects may compound these difficulties.

ECG definitions of myocardial ischaemia

In the absence of left ventricular hypertrophy (LVH) and left bundle branch block (LBBB):

ST elevation

ST elevation from J point in two contiguous leads with the cut off points: ≥0.2mV in men and 0.15mV in women in leads V2–3 and/or ≥0.15mV in any other leads.

ST depression and T wave changes

New horizontal or downsloping depression ≥0.05Mv in two contiguous leads; and/or T wave inversion in ≥0.1mV in two contiguous leads with prominent R wave or R/S >1.

Contiguous leads mean lead groups such as
- Anterior leads V1–6
- Inferior leads II, III, aVF
- Lateral/apical leads I and aVL.

Determinants of myocardial oxygen supply

- Anaemia (Hb <8.0g/dL) may predispose to myocardial ischaemia.
- Tachycardia: myocardial oxygen supply is determined by diastolic filling time.

- Hypotension: the diastolic BP and end-diastolic pressure gradient. The perfusion of the LV occurs in diastole while the RV can be perfused in both systole and diastole.
- Increased demand due to the use of inotropes such as adrenalin and dobutamine.

Myocardial oxygen demand is determined by heart rate (HR) and systolic BP which can be quantified as the rate pressure product. Therefore hypertension and tachycardias should be avoided. Myocardial ischaemia results from an imbalance between myocardial oxygen supply and demand.

Echocardiographic findings in myocardial ischaemia or infarction

A new regional wall-motion abnormality may indicate myocardial ischaemia or infarction. This may reflect the distribution of a particular coronary artery or be more global in character. There may also be global LV or RV systolic and/or diastolic dysfunction. In some cases, new mitral regurgitation or ventricular septal defect (VSD) may be identified.

Myocardial ischaemia can be induced even in the presence of normal coronary arteries.

Investigations in suspected myocardial ischaemia

- 12-lead ECG
- Echocardiogram
- Review of operative intervention.

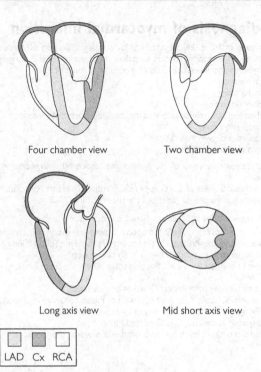

Four chamber view   Two chamber view

Long axis view   Mid short axis view

LAD Cx RCA

Figure 5.1 Typical regions of myocardium perfused by each of the major coronary arteries to the left ventricle. Other patterns occur as a result of normal anatomical variations or coronary disease with collateral flow. LAD: left anterior descending; Cx: circumflex; RCA: right coronary artery. Reprinted from the *Journal of the American Society of Echocardiography*, 12, 10, Shanewise, J. et al., 'ASE/SCA guidelines for performing a comprehensive intraoperative multiplane transesophageal echocardiography examination: recommendations of the American Society of Echocardiography Council for Intraoperative Echocardiography and the Society of Cardiovascular Anesthesiologists Task Force for Certification in Perioperative Transesophageal Echocardiography', pp. 884–900, Copyright 1999, with permission from American Society of Echocardiography and Elsevier.

The diagnosis of myocardial infarction

The diagnosis of MI is difficult after cardiac surgery. Elevation of cardiac biomarkers such as troponin occurs to various degrees after cardiac surgery due to myocardial cell necrosis. This may occur as a result of:

- Surgical trauma
- Cardiac handling
- Coronary dissection
- Global or regional ischaemia due to inadequate myocardial protection and reperfusion injury
- Damage from oxygen free radicals
- Inadequate revascularization.

However, major elevations of biomarkers are associated with worsened prognosis.

The European Society of Cardiology (ESC)/American Heart Association (AHA) consensus guidelines redefined the types of MI in 2007.

Type 5 myocardial infarction (post cardiac surgery)

In CABG with normal baseline troponin values, elevation of cardiac bio-markers above the 99th percentile upper reference limit (URL) is indicative of perioperative myocardial necrosis. By convention:

- Increases in biomarkers >5 × 99th percentile during the first 72 hours after CABG:
  - plus either new pathological Q waves or new LBBB
  - or angiographically new graft occlusion or native coronary occlusion
  - or imaging evidence of new loss of myocardium have been designated as defining CABG-related MI.
- Elevated biomarkers levels are associated with a worse prognosis.

Management: general principles

Initial interventions are targeted at reducing ischaemia

- Control tachycardia HR <100bpm.
- Normalize BP: MAP 70–100mmHg.
- Reduce end-diastolic pressures with vasodilators such as glyceryl trinitrate (GTN).
- If hypertensive reduce inotropes.
- Correct hypotension.
- This may be due to hypovolaemia or ischaemia-induced myocardial dysfunction or vasodilation.
- Beware: inotropes may increase myocardial oxygen demand.
- Administer aspirin if bleeding is controlled.

If simple measures are ineffective:

- Consider the insertion of an IABP early as it is beneficial to the supply/demand balance and may allow weaning of inotropes.
- Consider surgical intervention with re-exploration if malfunctioning graft is suspected.
- Emergency coronary angiography with possible percutaneous coronary intervention (PCI).

If the diagnosis of MI is established in the postoperative period, therapy is similar to the management of patients in a non-cardiac setting with the exception that thrombolysis is contraindicated in the postoperative period due to the risks of bleeding.

MI can be complicated with:
- Arrhythmias
- Cardiogenic shock
- Organ dysfunction
- VSD
- Papillary muscle rupture and severe mitral regurgitation (MR).

Supportive therapy is targeted on the following aims:
- Re-establish coronary perfusion if possible
- Maintain systemic perfusion
- Avoid organ dysfunction
- Treat arrhythmias
- Identify and treat any complications
- Secondary prevention with aspirin and statins.

Cardiogenic shock may require treatment with:
- IABP
- Inotropes
- Vasodilators such as milrinone
- Ventricular assist device (VAD).

Key point

In myocardial ischaemia, every effort should be made to identify remediable causes early as technical issues with coronary grafts may be amenable to intervention by reoperation or PCI.

Bleeding management

Introduction

Cardiac surgery is responsible for 15% of all blood products used in the UK.

All cardiac patients have some drainage from the chest drains postoperatively. This is variable in quantity and blood content with wide variations between units depending on individual protocols for:

- Bypass circuit types including oxygenators, filters, and cannulae
- Heparin and its reversal
- Perfusion temperatures
- Bypass duration.

Bleeding may be of surgical or non-surgical types and often causes haemodynamic instability and/or cardiac tamponade. These effects and subsequent transfusion are associated with multiple negative outcomes and an ↑ mortality rate.

Excessive bleeding is difficult to define and definitions vary. A good rule of thumb is:

- >300mL in first hour
- >200mL/hour for 2 consecutive hours
- >150mL/hour for 4 consecutive hours.

Blood may accumulate in open pleural cavities and appear intermittently in significant aliquots.

It could be anticipated that up to 20% of patients may breach local protocols and that approximately 5% will require repeat sternotomy. It is often difficult to distinguish surgical haemorrhage from true coagulopathic bleeding, but left untreated surgical bleeding will progress to coagulopathy. Early re-sternotomy may limit exposure to unnecessary blood and factor replacement.

Identified patient factors for excessive bleeding include:

- Age >70 years
- Preoperative anaemia
- Female gender
- Small body size/low BMI
- Urgent or emergency status.

Cardiac surgery and cardiopulmonary bypass

Cardiac surgery provides a unique set of circumstances to affect coagulation and fibrinolysis. The interaction of blood with non-endothelial surfaces in CPB releases tissue factors which activates cellular and humoral mechanisms; including the coagulation cascade, complement and fibrinolytic systems. Platelets and leucocytes are thereafter stimulated leading to the clinical effects of oedema, tissue injury, hyperfibrinolysis and a consumptive coagulopathy.

Excessive postoperative non-surgical bleeding is related to platelet dysfunction, impaired coagulation, and ↑ fibrinolysis.

Technique and disease-specific issues include:

- Systemic heparinization
- Normovolaemic haemodilution with dilution of platelets and coagulation factors

- Substantive transfusion of salvaged blood may increase dilutional effects
- Hypothermia which continues into immediate perioperative period and increases with bypass duration
- Antithrombotic drug therapy
- Antiplatelet therapy
- Warfarin therapy—inhibits vitamin K-dependent synthesis of factors II, VII, IX, X.

Excessive bleeding

Up to 5% of cardiac surgical patients will require re-sternotomy in the early postoperative period. Stable patients with higher than expected blood loss may return to theatre but unstable patients are best managed in the ITU environment (Fig. 6.1).

Bleeding may be:
- Overt with rapid or ongoing haemorrhage:
  - >300mL in first hour
  - >200mL/hour for 2 consecutive hours
  - >150mL/hour for 4 consecutive hours
- Concealed presenting as haemodynamic instability and ongoing requirement for transfusion:
  - *Beware pleural collections*, consider chest X-ray (CXR) and echo examination of the pleural spaces
- Localized to the pericardial cavity and present with cardiac tamponade. See ▢ Cardiac tamponade, p. 46.

If untreated, bleeding and its complications will progress to cardiac arrest.

Ongoing assessment and proactive management are important to avoid the additional complications of coagulopathy and massive transfusion.

The decision to re-open is complex. The patient's preoperative condition including recent anticoagulation, the duration of bypass, and any surgical difficulties in theatre all inform the decision of whether to perform re-sternotomy.

Patients who require re-exploration are more likely to have the complications of:
- Renal failure
- Sepsis
- Atrial fibrillation
- Prolonged mechanical ventilation
- ↑ hospital stay
- ↑ overall mortality.

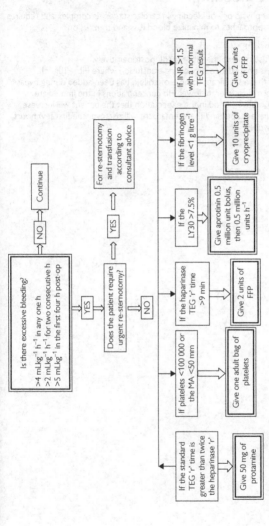

Figure 6.1 Management of coagulopathy. Reproduced from P Diprose, 'Reducing allogeneic transfusion in cardiac surgery: a randomized double-blind placebo-controlled trial of antifibrinolytic therapies used in addition to intra-operative cell salvage', *British Journal of Anaesthesia*, 2005, 94, 3, pp. 271–278, by permission of The Board of Management and Trustees of the British Journal of Anaesthesia and Oxford University Press.

Overt bleeding

The pathophysiology of bleeding in cardiac surgery is complex and requires multiple approaches to minimize blood loss and transfusions.

Transfusion

- Transfuse to keep the Hb >7g/dL postoperatively.
- There is no evidence supporting transfusion where Hb >10g/dL.
- Given that a significant volume of colloid has been added during bypass, it is normal to tolerate lower Hb concentrations in the immediate postoperative period in the expectation that the patient will increase their urine output and the haematocrit will rise over the first few hours post bypass.

Concealed bleeding

Patients may have concealed haemorrhage if they require more volume replacement than anticipated in the first 2–4 hours after surgery. They are more likely to be tachycardic and BP will improve with transfusion of volume, but then fall again. Red cells will be required to maintain the haemoglobin >7g/dL:

- It is important to know if the pleurae are open following surgery, as blood may collect in the pleural spaces. A CXR will show ↑ opacification if there is a pleural collection.
- The peritoneum may be breached at sternotomy, and may become a reservoir for concealed haemorrhage.
- Both the upper and lower GI tract may conceal haemorrhage, and should be considered if the source of bleeding cannot be identified.
- Consider retroperitoneal haemorrhage if an IABP has been inserted.
- Persisting bleeding from the legs may occur if vein has been harvested during surgery. Inspection of the legs should be included in the search for hidden haemorrhage.

Cardiac tamponade

Cardiac tamponade is the clinical syndrome when blood collects in the pericardial space reducing ventricular filling and causing haemodynamic compromise. This can be produced with rapid accumulations of <150mL.

Physiology

Normal cardiac filling is bimodal:

- Initially venous return increases with the onset of ventricular contraction and subsequent decrease in intrapericardial pressure (x descent of CVP).
- Later RV filling in diastole with opening of tricuspid valve (y descent). This is diminished or absent in tamponade.

Diastolic filling is diminished when the transmural distending pressures are insufficient to overcome the intrapericardial pressures. Venous return is impeded with right atrial and ventricular collapse. Output is initially maintained by tachycardia. The compliance of the pulmonary vascular bed causes blood to pool in the venous circulation at the expense of LV filling and CO.

Whilst the pericardium may be reconstituted after valve surgery, this is rarely carried out in coronary revascularization. Despite the large potential space if the pleura is opened, localized tamponade on the right atrium can have significant haemodynamic effects.

Mediastinal chest drains are inserted as standard postoperative practice. However, they may occlude despite measures to maintain patency.

Early detection and treatment of cardiac tamponade is crucial in postoperative management. It often coexists in complex patients with low output states.

Classical features include:

- ↑ HR
- Pulsus paradoxus (exaggerated decrease in systolic BP in inspiration). May be 20–40mmHg in tamponade but difficult to diagnose in hypotensive or ventilated patients
- ↑ jugular venous pressure (JVP)/CVP
- ECG—low voltage complexes or electrical alternans.
- ↓ BP
- ↓ CO
- ↓ urinary output
- Cardiomegaly on CXR.

Atypical features:

- Failure to rewarm
- Unexpected dysrhythmias
- Lower than expected CO
- Metabolic/lactic acidosis.

Diagnosis may be difficult especially in patients with low output states. Echocardiography is a useful adjunct to diagnosis but a high index of clinical suspicion should always be present in:

- High-risk patients
- When higher than average mediastinal losses suddenly diminish
- Failure of patients to progress as expected.

Echocardiography

Cardiac tamponade cannot be excluded with echocardiography. Classical features include:
- Echo-free space ant/post/global
- Diastolic collapse of RV free wall (parasternal short axis at aortic valve)
- Late diastolic compression/collapse of RA.

Difficulties

- Poor transthoracic access due to sternal wound/drains/pacing wires
- Organized clot may be difficult to distinguish from myocardium and mediastinal structures
- Ubiquitous left pleural effusion.

Differential diagnosis

- Tension pneumothorax
- Hypovolaemic shock
- Acute right heart failure
- MI
- Congestive cardiac failure.

Further reading

Diprose P, Herbertson MJ, O'Shaughnessy D, Deakin CD, Gill RS. Reducing allogenic transfusion in cardiac surgery: a randomized double blind placebo controlled trial of anti-fibrinolytic therapy used in addition to intra-operative cell salvage. *BJA* 2005;94(3):271–8.

Society of Thoracic Surgeons Blood Conservation Guideline Task Force, Ferraris VA, Ferraris SP, Saha SP, Hessel EA 2nd, Haan CK, et al. Peri-operative Blood Transfusion and Blood Conservation in Cardiac Surgery: the Society of Thoracic Surgeons and Society of Cardiovascular Anaesthesiologists Clinical Practice Guideline. *Ann Thor Surg* 2007;83:S27–86.

Chapter 7

Postoperative hypotension

Introduction

Hypotension is a common occurrence in up to 75% of patients in the early postoperative period after cardiac surgery. As the BP is easy to measure it is used as a surrogate for impaired tissue perfusion. In fact the BP and the flow are equally important to regional perfusion.

There are no global accepted definitions for hypotension, however, for the purposes of this chapter we shall define hypotension as a fall in the systolic BP to <90mmHg or the MAP to <65mmHg.

An understanding of the relationship between BP and flow is essential. In many ways the MAP is a more important measure than the systolic pressure which is more influenced by damping and vascular impedance and is less directly linked to flow.

When assessing a critical care patient, the perfusion pressure should be calculated by subtracting CVP from the MAP. Patients with high CVPs require higher MAP to achieve an adequate perfusion pressure.

The perfusion pressure is directly proportional to the product of the cardiac index (CI) and the systemic vascular resistance (SVR) and may be manipulated by influencing these indices by pharmacological or mechanical interventions.

Autoregulation across a vascular bed results in stable flow across a range of MAPs. In the cerebral circulation this is typically from a cerebral perfusion pressure (CPP) of 50–150mmHg. The autoregulation curve may be shifted to the right in various diseased states such as long-standing hypertension or when autoregulation is impaired.

In the assessment of hypotensive patients in the postoperative period after cardiac surgery, it is important to know what the BP was before surgery as this acts as a baseline.

Also other indices of perfusion must be considered alongside the BP such as:
- Urine output
- Arterial H$^+$
- Plasma lactate
- Mixed venous saturation.

Goals for MAP should be set on an individual patient basis taking into account preoperative factors such as a history of hypertension and baseline ventricular function.

Management of hypotension: general principles

Diagnosis

Hypotension is commonly a result of the following (see Table 7.1):
- Preload reduction (hypovolaemia)
- Impaired cardiac function
- Reduced afterload (vasoplegia).

Table 7.1 Early postoperative hypotension: the common causes, helpful investigations, and typical interventions

Diagnosis	MAP	CVP	HR	Treatment	Investigation
Hypovolaemia	––	––	++	Fluid challenge	Echo
Myocardial failure	––	++	++/0	Inotropes, IABP, VAD	Echo, PAFC, 12-lead ECG
Tamponade	––	++	++/0	Surgical reopening	Echo, CXR
Tension Pneumothorax	––	++	+/–	Pleural drain	CXR
Vasoplegia	––	+/–	+/–	Noradrenaline, vasopressin, methylene blue	Echo, PAFC

Preload

- Maintain preload
- Assess response to fluid challenge (see algorithm in Fig. 7.1)
- Beware concealed blood loss.

Preload may be difficult to assess. The absolute CVP is a poor measure of preload and the dynamic response of the MAP, HR, CVP, and other indirect indices of perfusion to a fluid challenge may be better.

An ↑ pulse pressure variation may indicate hypovolaemia and suggest volume responsiveness.

In patients who are unresponsive to fluid challenge, more information may be necessary to guide treatments.

A full assessment of the past medical history, ventricular function, conduct of the operation including any clinical difficulties in theatre, and clinical examination often raises suspicion of a possible likely cause.

A bedside echocardiogram can help differentiate between hypovolaemia, impaired cardiac function and vasoplegia. The insertion of a pulmonary artery flotation catheter (PAFC) will help differentiate between low CO syndrome and vasoplegia.

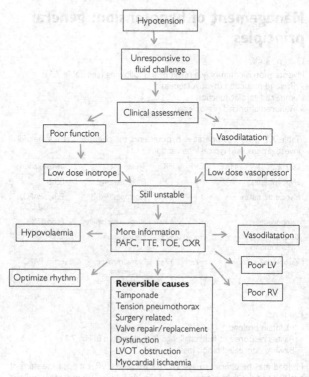

Figure 7.1 Management algorithm for hypotension post cardiac surgery.

Reversible causes of hypotension

Dysrhythmia

Changes in heart rhythm can precipitate hypotension. The heart rate and rhythm is assessed and corrected if possible. When tachydysrhythmias are associated with profound hypotension and compromised perfusion, DC cardioversion should be considered. Bradycardias may be treated by pacing if epicardial pacing wires have been placed during surgery. Loss of atrioventricular (AV) synchrony may have a disproportionate effect in patients with impaired ventricular function and/or diastolic dysfunction and LV hypertrophy. DDD pacing may be beneficial.

Hypovolaemia and tamponade

Excessive bleeding will cause hypotension and can be diagnosed by ↑ surgical drainage (>200mL/hour).

Beware of concealed haemorrhage as this may occur particularly when the pleural spaces have been opened. A clinical examination and a CXR will identify a significant haemothorax.

Hypotension may be a result of cardiac tamponade which is a clinical diagnosis. The hallmarks of cardiac tamponade are:
• Hypotension
• Tachycardia
• Raised CVP
• Poor perfusion (delayed capillary filling and adverse trending of perfusion indices).

When in doubt an echocardiogram can confirm the diagnosis (see 📖 Management of hypotension: general principles, p. 51).

Specific surgery-related causes of hypotension

• Regional myocardial ischaemia
• Valve replacement or repair dysfunction
• LV outflow tract (LVOT) obstruction after replacement or repair.

An index of suspicion must be maintained for the recognition of reversible causes of hypotension which are specific to the cardiac surgical procedure.

Poor myocardial performance may be due to regional myocardial ischaemia. This may be suspected if there are ECG changes in the territory of a single coronary artery and/or matching new wall-motion abnormality on echocardiography. Suspected myocardial ischaemia may indicate a technical issue with a CABG and be an indication for reoperation or coronary angiography and PCI.

If, after valve repair or replacement, resistant hypotension is problematic this may indicate a failure of the operative procedure. Valvular annuloplasty rings can become dehisced and leaflets of mechanical valves may be stuck. These can be diagnosed by transoesophageal echocardiography (TOE) and reoperation may be indicated.

After mitral valve repair or aortic valve replacement, LVOT obstruction may cause early hypotension. These should be excluded by echocardiography; however, generally an index of suspicion will be present from intraoperative echocardiographic findings and this should have been handed over to the cardiac intensive care staff on admission.

Features of low cardiac output syndrome (CI <2.2L/min)

- Low CO
- Cold peripheries
- Impaired capillary refilling
- Hypotension
- Raised H^+ and lactate
- Low urine output
- Low mixed venous saturation (<60%).

Treatment

- Optimize HR/usually 80–90bpm
- Rhythm (aim for normal sinus rhythm (NSR) and AV synchrony)
- Optimize preload
- Address any reversible causes
- Pharmacological support: inotropes: catecholamines, phosphodiesterase inhibitors, calcium sensitization
- Optimize and normalize biochemical milieu (K^+, Ca^{2+}, H^+)
- Improve oxygen carrying by correcting anaemia
- Mechanical support: IABP or VAD
- Reduced afterload.

Vasoplegic syndrome

Vasoplegic syndrome occurs in 8.8% of cardiac surgical patients in the early postoperative period. It can be defined by the presence of the following five criteria:

- Hypotension MAP <50mmHg
- Low filling pressures: CVP <5mmHg; pulmonary capillary wedge pressure (PCWP) <10mmHg
- High or normal CI >2.5L/min/m^2
- Low peripheral resistance, SVR <800dyne/sec/cm^5
- A vasopressor requirement.

At-risk groups

- Transplants
- Poor ejection fraction (EF)%
- Use of angiotensin-converting enzyme (ACE) inhibitors.

Typically associated with:

- CPB
- Long bypass runs
- Systemic inflammatory response syndrome (SIRS)
- ↑ use of constrictors on CPB.

Treatment
- Confirm diagnosis with echo and/or PAFC
- Minimize use of vasodilators (GTN, milrinone, and sedation)
- *Pharmacological vasoconstriction:*
  - Noradrenaline: infusion starting at 0.05mcg/kg/min
  - Vasopressin: infusion starting at 2IU/hour (working range 0–4IU/hour)
  - Methylene blue: methylene blue comes as 1% (10mg/mL). Bolus dose 1.5mg/kg. Make up to 50mL with sterile water and infuse over 20–30 minutes.

Tension pneumothorax

Clinical signs include:
- Hypotension
- High airway pressures
- Arterial desaturation
- Air leak into drains
- Unequal air entry on auscultation
- Evidence of tracheal shift away from pneumothorax.

If the patient is relatively stable then time can be taken to perform a CXR which will be diagnostic. In extremis, if clinical suspicion exists, a drainage cannula should be inserted into the 2nd intercostal space to relieve the tension. Once stabilized, an intercostal drain should be inserted under sterile conditions.

Further reading

Levin RL, Degrange MA, Bruno GF, Del Mazo CD, Taborda DJ, Griotti JJ, et al. Methylene blue reduces mortality and morbidity in vasoplegic patients after cardiac surgery. *Ann Thorac Surg* 2004;77(2):496–9.

Glucose, lactate, and acid–base

Introduction

Acid–base biochemistry, lactate metabolism, and even glucose metabolism are complex. In an individual patient it may be difficult to interpret with certainty the precise mechanisms underlying the measured trends. Nevertheless, these measurements are useful as indicators of potential physiological derangement, as guides to treatment, and as indicators of prognosis.

Despite the underlying complexity, a pragmatic approach extracts most of the immediate clinical value from the data with remarkably little mental effort.

Acid–base biochemistry

Overview

Hydrogen ion concentration in living tissue is tightly controlled because small changes in hydrogen ion concentration can have large qualitative and quantitative changes on a myriad of metabolic reactions. Plasma hydrogen ion concentration, which equates to extracellular fluid hydrogen ion concentration, is the only hydrogen ion concentration amenable to easy measurement. However this reflects only one physiological compartment and in particular, does not give reliable information about what is happening intracellularly.

pH is a traditional notation for hydrogen ion concentration that derives from the physical sciences and has become embedded in biological culture largely through historical custom. It is the negative logarithm of the actual hydrogen ion concentration and is useful for describing changes across large ranges. It is a non-linear scale. Hydrogen ion concentration $[H^+]$ is better for describing changes in the relevant clinical range.

The hydrogen ion concentration in an aqueous solution reflects the degree of dissociation of water. It is influenced by dissolved ions, by temperature and by buffers.

There are two common ways of conceptualizing the control of hydrogen ions in biological solutions. These are the traditional Henderson–Hasselbalch or bicarbonate-centred framework, and the Stewart (strong ion) hypothesis. In practice and mathematically these descriptions are equivalent. Strong ion theory is useful because it provides an immediate conceptual explanation for the clinical importance of chloride ions and other phenomena such as dilution acidosis. It does not, however, lend itself to easy calculation and the verity of its claims to provide insights into the causal mechanisms of hydrogen ion concentration remains debatable and experimentally unproven.

Stewart hypothesis

The hydrogen ion concentration of an aqueous biological solution is determined only by three variables from which it may be derived by a fourth-order polynomial equation. These are: [SID], $[A_{TOT}]$, and PCO_2, where [SID], the strong ion difference is the difference in the net charge concentration (mmol/L) of the fixed cations and anions fully dissociated in solution, $[A_{TOT}]$ is the concentration of partially dissociated weak acids (albumin, other serum proteins and inorganic phosphate), and PCO_2 is the partial pressure of dissolved CO_2.

Since [SID] is given by

$$[SID] = [Na^+] + [K^+] + [Ca^{2+}] + [Mg^{2+}] - [Cl^-] - [other strong anions]$$

It is easy to see (at least qualitatively) how hyperchloraemia (relative to [Na^+]) is associated with acidosis and hypochloraemia is associated with alkalosis. Similarly it can be seen that changes in plasma volume due to dehydration or dilution will change the absolute size of the strong ion difference with resultant effects on plasma [H^+].

Blood gas analysis

Clinical blood gas analysis is based on the bicarbonate-centred approach. It assumes plasma acidity is determined by the concentration of volatile acid (CO_2) and the concentration of non-volatile acids (all other acids apart from CO_2).

An acid tendency caused by excess CO_2 is termed a *respiratory* acidosis. An alkaline tendency caused by lack of CO_2 is termed a *respiratory* alkalosis. Similarly the effects of excess or deficiency of non-volatile acids are termed *metabolic* acidosis and alkalosis respectively. These effects may compensate for each other and a combination of metabolic and respiratory effects is often present. Resultant changes in the actual [H^+] are termed acidaemia (high [H^+]) and alkalaemia (low [H^+]).

An effective approach to blood gas analysis may be based on three key variables: [H^+], SBE (the standard base excess), and PCO_2

Respiratory acidosis is caused by accumulation of CO_2 in the plasma. CO_2 is acidic because it forms carbonic acid:

$$CO_2 + H_2O = H_2CO_3 = H^+ + HCO_3^- \quad \text{(Eqn 8.1)}$$

The PCO_2 defines the size of the respiratory acidosis or alkalosis. High PCO_2 indicates respiratory acidosis, low PCO_2 indicates respiratory alkalosis.

CO_2 is the end product of metabolism and is excreted through the lungs. Excess CO_2 thus occurs as a result of ↑ production or ↓ clearance. The commonest cause of ↓ clearance in the early postoperative period is opioid–mediated respiratory depression (this contrasts with the sick patient who has been ventilated for a longer period where mechanical respiratory insufficiency and poor gas exchange are likely to be important factors.) The treatment is adjustment of analgesia ± temporary prolongation of mechanical support. The commonest cause of ↑ production in the early postoperative period is shivering.

Practice point

Consider shivering as a cause of respiratory acidosis in the re-warming patient. Treat with pethidine (25mg IV repeated once if necessary) escalating to ↑ sedation in the intubated patient and, if still problematic, neuromuscular blockade (only in anaesthetized patients).

Metabolic acidosis

SBE, the standard base excess, defines the size of the *metabolic* acidosis or alkalosis.

SBE is the amount of acid or alkali required to titrate the extracellular fluid [H^+] back to normal in the presence of a normal pCO_2. The term 'standard' refers to the fact that the value is corrected for the buffering effect of haemoglobin so as to estimate the base excess for whole body extracellular fluid (ECF) rather than the base excess of the plasma in the sample. By convention, base excess is described as mEq/L of alkali so a negative base excess is an acidosis.

The key importance of a metabolic acidosis is in the diagnosis and treatment of the underlying cause. Important causes of metabolic acidosis in the early postoperative period include low CO (often accompanied by high lactate) and renal insufficiency (failure of H^+ excretion: lactate is usually normal). A transient lactic acidosis may develop in the first few postoperative hours in a patient who is otherwise well, particularly in patients receiving exogenous adrenaline.

Treatment of metabolic acidosis

Direct treatment of metabolic acidosis by alkali administration in the form of bicarbonate remains controversial. Clinical evidence is lacking. Theoretical arguments are contradictory. A pragmatic approach may be taken:

- Make a careful search for and manage the underlying cause.
- Leave moderate degrees of abnormality (up to about base excess −10) to self-correct.
- In the acidotic patient with acute cardiac decompensation, administering bicarbonate to partially correct the acidosis *may* increase cardiac contractile force and the efficacy of exogenous inotropes and vasopressors, which might contribute to a virtuous circle of recovery. Give bicarbonate in aliquots of 50–100mmol titrated against blood gas measurements, *while monitoring for volume overload*. In the ventilated patient, simultaneously increase ventilation to rigorously maintain normocapnia, or mild hypocapnia. CO_2 diffuses freely across cell membranes and the CO_2 load associated with the neutralization of the carbonic acid (see Eqn 8.1) may otherwise worsen intracellular acidosis. The total amount of bicarbonate required to correct an existing acidosis can be calculated from:

$$\text{Dose (mEq)} = 0.3 \times \text{weight(Kg)} \times \text{SBE(mEq/L)} \quad \text{(Eqn 8.2)}$$

Most clinicians would regard total correction as too aggressive.

Temperature correction. Blood gas and acid base results should be inter-preted at 37°C rather than corrected for the patient's actual temperature (analogous to alpha stat pH management during bypass).

The patient's acid–base status in the immediate postoperative period will reflect fluid management during theatre. An acidic pump prime will leave a small residual metabolic acidosis.

Mixed effects

Metabolic and respiratory acidosis may coexist, e.g. in the unconscious or under-ventilated patient with cardiogenic shock. In this case their effects on [H^+] will be additive and there will be an acidaemia. The metabolic and respiratory effects may be in opposite directions as the body attempts to normalize the [H^+], e.g. in the case of prolonged type 2 respiratory failure. In this case the compensation is almost always incomplete and the [H^+] indi-cates the direction of the primary abnormality, e.g. if the [H^+] is high there is a primary acidosis with a compensatory respiratory alkalosis. However the main clue is usually provided by the clinical history.

Blood gas results and acid–base chemistry should always be interpreted in the light of the clinical history.

Lactate

Metabolite lactate is formed from pyruvate which is a normal product of metabolism.

Lactate metabolism and its control is complex both at a whole-body level and a cellular level. Changes in concentration may reflect changes in production or changes in removal. A raised plasma lactate is not thought to be harmful in itself. Lactate is formed during anaerobic metabolism in muscles and thus ↑ lactate concentrations may reflect inadequate tissue perfusion, for instance, caused by low CO. However, other causes of raised lactate in the immediate postoperative period include ↑ production due to β 2 receptor stimulation (adrenaline) and the systemic inflammatory response (cytokine-mediated stimulation).

A raised or rising lactate should thus precipitate a careful diagnostic review for signs of circulatory insufficiency but, by itself, is not diagnostic of an adverse situation. It is usefully reassuring if the lactate concentration is normal.

A high lactate (>3mmol/L) at entry to intensive care is associated with a raised mortality in observational studies.

Practice point

Switching a patient away from an adrenaline-based inotrope regimen may normalize a raised lactate

Glucose

Blood glucose concentration rises during and after cardiac surgery due to stress response and exogenous beta stimulation.

There is no strong evidence for treating blood glucose after cardiac surgery differently than in other critical care situations. Glucose should be kept in the range 3.5–10.0mmol/L using continuous infusion of insulin adjusted according to a protocol. The main danger of tighter control is hypoglycaemia.

The causal relationship between high blood glucose and lactataemia is unclear.

An important feature of glucose control is keeping input constant. Enteral or parenteral feeding should thus be administered continuously over 24 hours. If feeding is interrupted for any reason insulin infusions should be stopped or reduced and glucose concentration monitored closely.

Terminology

Whole blood glucose concentrations differ from plasma values, because the concentration in whole red cells is lower due to their high lipid content. Whole blood concentrations can be converted to plasma concentrations by multiplying by 1.11 at normal haematocrit. Since 2001, all laboratory and point-of-care resting values should be reported as plasma concentrations regardless of the actual method of measurement.

Further reading

Grogono AW. *Acid-Base Tutorial*. Available at: ℜ <http://www.acid-base.com>.
Kurtz I, Kraut J, Ornekian V, Nguyen MK. Acid-base analysis: a critique of the Stewart and bicarbonate-centered approaches. *Am J Physiol Renal Physiol* 2008;294:F1009–F1031.

Postoperative medications

Postoperative medications

Postoperative critical care involves getting the basics right, attention to detail, and avoidance of omissions. Most postoperative medications are prescribed according to a standard protocol (see example protocol in Table 9.1). Cardiac surgical patients are commonly on numerous medications some of which must be continued into the postoperative period and others which should be stopped. This chapter covers the common drugs prescribed in the postoperative period after cardiac surgery.

Antibiotic prophylaxis

- Prophylaxis against surgical site infection is routinely continued into the postoperative period. Local policies will vary. These are generally not continued beyond 24 hours after surgery. See ▣ Antimicrobial therapy, p. 34.

Stress ulcer prophylaxis

- Prophylaxis is essential in patients mechanically ventilated for >48 hours.
- The combination of major surgery, hypoperfusion, systemic anticoagulation, and potential coagulopathy makes patients high risk for development of stress ulcers—prophylaxis is started preoperatively.

Electrolytes

- Hypokalaemia and hypomagnesaemia are common in the postoperative period and put patients at ↑ risk of arrhythmia.
- Plasma potassium should be maintained >4.0mmol/L, or >4.5mmol/L if arrhythmias are present.
- IV magnesium is a safe and effective antiarrhythmic agent and is commonly used to prevent postoperative arrhythmias:
  - Caution: rapid infusion of magnesium can cause hypotension and bradycardia.

Antiemetics

- Should be available as required to treat PONV. Postoperative ileus and opiates may also cause PONV.

Shivering

- Shivering increases oxygen demand and should be avoided.
- Can be due to hypothermia requiring resedation and further warming.
- Postoperative shivering often responds to pethidine.

Glucose control

- Hyperglycaemia is common after cardiac surgery and associated with ↑ mortality and complications in patients both with and without diabetes mellitus.
- Blood glucose should be controlled by using a continuous, IV insulin infusion, e.g. by sliding scale, to maintain median blood glucose control between 3.5mmol/L and 10mmol/L. Perioperative blood glucose control after cardiac surgery reduces mortality:
  - Caution: avoid hypoglycaemia.

Deep venous thrombosis prophylaxis

- Patients are at risk for DVT due to the procoagulant effect of major surgery, immobility, and the loss of saphenous veins/bandaging of limbs.
- Subcutaneous low-molecular-weight heparin (LMWH) is delayed until postoperative day 1 because of the risks of bleeding associated with cardiopulmonary bypass and cardiac surgery:
  - e.g. dalteparin 5000IU SC once daily.

Arrhythmia (atrial fibrillation) prophylaxis

- Early postoperative administration of β-blockers in patients without contraindications is standard therapy to reduce the incidence and/or clinical sequelae of atrial fibrillation. (Usually started on postoperative day 1 in patients not receiving inotropes—see 📖 Secondary prevention, p. 70.)
- Amiodarone is effective prophylaxis for high-risk patients with contraindications to β-blockers.

Table 9.1 Example protocol for postoperative prescribing on the day of surgery

Sedation and analgesia	
Propofol	0–5mcg/mL IV by target controlled infusion
Paracetamol	1g IV 6-hourly
Morphine	Nurse-controlled IV boluses until extubated then 5–10mg SC PRN up to hourly
Antibiotic prophylaxis	
Flucloxacillin	1g IV 6-hourly (for 3 doses)
Gentamicin	Single dose only at induction
Stress ulcer prophylaxis	
Ranitidine	50mg IV 8-hourly until extubated
Electrolytes	
Potassium chloride	12.5–25mmol IV PRN by infusion
Magnesium sulphate	10–20mmol IV PRN by infusion
Antiemetics	
Ondansetron	4mg IV PRN up to 8-hourly
Control of shivering	
Pethidine	25–50mg IV PRN
Glucose control	
Actrapid® insulin	Actrapid® 50IU in 50mL by sliding scale

Note: This table represents normal practice in the author's institution but should not be considered absolute. Refer to local guidelines.

Postoperative medication following coronary bypass/valve surgery

Medication following coronary bypass surgery

Prevention of coronary graft thrombosis
- Aspirin is the drug of choice for prophylaxis against early saphenous vein graft (SVG) thrombosis and should be given 6 hours post-operatively or as soon as bleeding has ceased:
  - e.g. aspirin 300mg PR (continued at 75mg PO daily long term).
  - The benefit of postoperative aspirin on SVG patency is lost when started >48 hours after surgery.
- Clopidogrel is an acceptable alternative to aspirin for the maintenance of graft patency in patients intolerant of aspirin:
  - Superiority over aspirin has not been established.
  - Patients on long-term dual therapy (aspirin and clopidogrel), e.g. stents, should have the dual therapy recommenced.

Secondary prevention (postoperative day 1 onwards)
- It is indicated to start and continue β-blocker therapy in all patients after MI, ACS, or LV dysfunction, unless contraindicated (see ERC/EACTS guidelines, 📖 Further reading, p. 71).
- β-blockers should be recommenced or considered for all patients without contraindications:
  - Contraindications: asthma or bronchospasm, HR <60bpm or pacemaker-dependent, BP <100mmHg systolic, or on inotropes.
  - Dose started low followed by upward dose titration.
  - e.g. bisoprolol 1.25mg PO daily.
- ACE inhibitors should be started and continued indefinitely in all patients with LVEF <40% and for those with hypertension, diabetes, or chronic kidney disease, unless contraindicated.
- ACE inhibitors should be gradually recommenced/considered in all patients (particularly patients with evidence of LV dysfunction):
  - Contraindications: acute or unstable renal impairment, BP <100mmHg systolic, or on inotropes.
  - e.g. ramipril 2.5mg PO daily.
- Statins should be recommenced or introduced in all patients:
  - Contraindications: acute liver disease, persistently abnormal liver function tests.
  - e.g. Simvastatin 40mg PO nocte.

Prevention of coronary graft spasm
- Radial artery grafts are particularly prone to spasm therefore vasodilators are commonly used:
  - e.g. glyceryl trinitrate 1–5mg/hour IV starting intraoperatively.
  - e.g. amlodipine 5mg PO daily continued for 3–6 months.

Medication following valve surgery

Prevention of valve thrombosis

- All patients with mechanical valves require anticoagulation.
- Bioprosthetic valves have an ↑ risk of thromboemboli during the first 3 months.
- Oral anticoagulation is recommended for the following situations:
  - Lifelong for all patients with mechanical valves irrespective of valve type or date of introduction.
  - Lifelong for patients with bioprostheses or mitral repair who have other indications for anticoagulation, e.g. atrial fibrillation and impaired LV function.
  - For the first 3 months, in all patients with bioprostheses or mitral valve repair involving the use of a prosthetic annuloplasty ring. (There is widespread use of aspirin as an alternative to anticoagulation for the first 3 months in patients with no other indications for anticoagulation.)
- Target INR depends on valve position, risk of thrombosis, and type of valve (see Table 9.2).
- Warfarin should be commenced on postoperative day 1 unless chest drains remain *in situ* for bleeding.

Table 9.2 Target INR following valve surgery

Mechanical aortic: no risk factors[a] —low/medium/high-risk valve[b]	2.5/3.0/3.5
Mechanical aortic: with risk factors[a] —low/medium/high-risk valve[b]	3.0/3.5/4.0
Mechanical mitral valve —low/medium/high-risk valve[b]	3.0 /3.5/4.0
Bioprosthesis: aortic—no risk factors[a]	Aspirin only
Bioprosthesis: aortic—risk factors[a]	2.5 (3 months)
Bioprosthesis: mitral	2.5 (3 months)

[a]Risk factors: atrial fibrillation, left atrium >50mm, ejection fraction <35%, additional valve replacements, hypercoagulability, history of thromboembolism.

[b]Valve risk: low risk: Medtronic Hall, St Jude, Carbomedics. Medium risk: bileaflet valves with insufficient data, Bjork–Shiley. High risk: Lillehei–Kaster, Omniscience, Starr–Edwards.

European Society of Cardiology. Recommendations for the management of patients after heart valve surgery. *Eur Heart J* 2005;26:2463–71

Further reading

Task Force on Myocardial Revascularization of the European Society of Cardiology (ESC) and the European Association for Cardio-Thoracic Surgery (EACTS), *et al*. Guidelines on myocardial revascularisation. *Eur Heart J* 2010;31:2501–55.

Preoperative medications

Continuing essential medications

Drugs for neurological disorders

Epilepsy
- Generalized seizures occurring in the perioperative period can increase morbidity and mortality, thus patients with pre-existing seizure disorders require anticonvulsant medications to be continued.
- Many antiepileptic drugs are available as a suspension that can be given via NG tube. Phenytoin, valproate, and levetiracetam are available parenterally. Carbamazepine can be given PR. There are no parenteral forms of gabapentin, topiramate, or lamotrigine—patients taking these medications in which the oral route is contraindicated require conversion to an alternative agent in consultation with a neurologist.

Parkinson's disease
- Liaison with specialist services is advised preoperatively.
- Adequate antiparkinsonian therapy is essential for satisfactory postoperative respiratory and bulbar muscle function.
- Dopaminergic drugs should be restarted as soon as possible postoperatively to reduce the risk of neuroleptic malignant syndrome (secondary to acute withdrawal).
- Many dopamine receptor agonists and levodopa/decarboxylase combinations can be administered via NG tube. Subcutaneous apomorphine or topical preparations of rotigotine (Neupro®) are available for patients in whom the oral route is contraindicated.
- Caution is required when prescribing other drugs—phenothiazines, butyrophenones, metoclopramide, and clonidine should be avoided.

Myasthenia gravis
- Careful management of anticholinesterase medication is essential to avoid myasthenic crisis and respiratory failure postoperatively.
- Anticholinesterases can be administered via NG tube and are usually restarted when the patient is haemodynamically stable, prior to weaning from mechanical ventilation and at the patient's usual dose.
- If the oral route is contraindicated, IV neostigmine is substituted for pyridostigmine at 1/30th the usual oral dose.
- Many drugs can worsen muscular weakness in myasthenia gravis. Aminoglycoside antibiotics should be avoided.
- Caution: patients with myasthenia gravis are often on corticosteroid therapy and will require additional supplementation.

Drugs for respiratory diseases

Inhaled bronchodilators and steroids should be continued in the intubated patient via nebulizer or metered dose inhaler attachment to the ventilator circuit. Beware tachycardia from β2 agonists.

Corticosteroids

Patients taking chronic glucocorticoid therapy require perioperative supplementation due to suppression of the hypothalamic–pituitary–adrenal axis.

- Patients taking >10mg prednisolone per day or who have stopped therapy <3 months ago are at risk.
- For major surgery, in addition to a bolus at induction of anaesthesia, patients require IV hydrocortisone 25–50mg 3 times a day for 48–72 hours postoperatively. Patients with high vasopressor requirement may require a prolonged course.

Restarting preoperative medications

Cardiovascular drugs

β-blockers, ACE inhibitors, and statins should be recommenced in patients with ischaemic heart disease (see 📖 Secondary prevention, p. 70). Antihypertensive, antianginal, and diuretic requirements may be different postoperatively and may not be required or can be titrated to effect.

Drugs for diabetes mellitus

Generally speaking, IV insulin infusions are continued until patients are eating and drinking when preoperative oral hypoglycaemics/SC insulins are recommenced:

- *Type 1 (and type 2 patients on insulin)*: long-acting insulins are withheld and total daily insulin requirement is administered as short-acting Actrapid® insulin (in 3–4 divided doses) until blood glucose is stable. Long-acting agents are then reintroduced.
- *Type 2*: caution should be exercised with certain drugs:
  - Sulfonylureas stimulate insulin secretion and may cause hypoglycaemia. Patients on high doses should start low and titrate upwards.
  - Metformin should not be restarted in patients with renal insufficiency, significant hepatic impairment, or congestive heart failure.
  - Thiazolidinediones should not be restarted in patients with congestive cardiac failure, problematic fluid retention, or liver function abnormalities.

Drugs for psychiatric disorders

Can generally be restarted on postoperative day 1. Caution is required with the following:

- Drugs prolonging QT-interval (particularly in association with class III antiarrhythmics).
- Selective serotonin reuptake inhibitors in combination with other drugs affecting serotonin levels (e.g. tramadol and ondansetron).

Sedation and analgesia

- See 📖 Pharmacology, p. 317.

Information handover and care planning

Introduction

Effective *communication* is an essential part of good team work which in turn helps set the scene for optimizing *patient safety*. Most human errors are not the result of poor technical knowledge or ability but are due instead to 'non-technical' aspects of performance such as communication.

Within a multidisciplinary team and between different tiers of a clinical team effective communication can be problematic, with differing communication styles complicated by hierarchical, ethnic, and gender influences.

Effective handover communication is vital at initial admission, staff changeovers, and on discharge from the cardiothoracic ICU. Within an intensive care environment a single patient's care may be 'handed over' within the multidisciplinary team over 15 times within any single 24-hour period.

Missing or incomplete information during admission or subsequent handover is a common cause of error and patient harm.

During the handover of information distractions or interruptions increase cognitive demands leading to inefficiency and an ↑ risk of error. This cognitive stress may be exacerbated when the patient is acutely unwell.

Good situation awareness and effective role and task allocation start with effective communication.

Handovers require the concise transfer of accurate and relevant patient information. This process can be aided by a *standardized written handover sheet* which details the objective clinical data. The *verbal handover* should include a short summary and highlight areas of clinical concern, outstanding tasks or plans, and take place between all health professionals of the same discipline or between different disciplines. There is no need to verbally repeat all the clinical data on the handover sheet as this will only increase the cognitive demands on the recipient.

One method of enabling effective handover is using a modified *SBAR tool*, developed by Kaiser Permanente, which is an easy focused way of setting expectations of a response that is appropriate and timely. SBAR encompasses the following:

- Situation:
  - Identify self, patient, bed space
  - Briefly state current issues and duration
- Background:
  - Diagnosis
  - Number of days in ICU
  - Current respiratory support
  - Current drug therapies
  - Relevant recent vital signs
  - Relevant lab results
- Assessment:
  - What do you think is going on?
  - What is your opinion?
- Response:
  - What actions are required?
  - Over what timescale?

ICU admission

Preparation for the patient's arrival
- ICU multidisciplinary team brief/planning and role allocation
- Equipment ready and checked
- Infusions prepared
- Handover sheet from theatre with relevant patient information including endotracheal tube (ETT) sizing, lines, inotropes, etc.

Patient arrival in ICU
- Patient monitoring transfer
- Patient support transfer (ventilator, inotropes, drain suction)
- Verbal handover:
  - One voice, *all* team watching and listening
  - No other tasks undertaken during handover
  - Clear and concise handover
  - SBAR technique
  - Handover sheet allows handover to be more subjective
- Encourage questions from all staff groups at end
- Summarize plans at end.

Post handover
- ICU team task allocation
- Appropriate investigations
- Multidisciplinary review of care plan.

Shift handover and ICU discharge

Written handover information can be used to provide the objective clinical data with the more subjective clinical impression and outstanding tasks being delineated by the following SBAR format.

- Situation:
  - Concise summary
  - Patient name
  - Primary diagnosis
  - Bed space
  - Age
  - Weight
- Background:
  - Diagnoses
  - Length of stay
  - Systems-based concise review
  - Current therapies
- Assessment:
  - Current issues in a system•based approach
- Response:
  - Outstanding tasks and timescale
  - Clinical teams involved.

Conclusion

Effective and efficient communication plays a central role if excellent multi-disciplinary care is to be delivered in any ICU.

Written and verbal communication can work hand in hand to allow such communication and care planning. The written data should provide the hard facts and the verbal handover, using an SBAR format, allows participants to focus on the pertinent facts, tasks, and areas of clinical concerns.

All disciplines in the ICU should continually be seeking to improve the care delivered. By taking a short period of time to think about how we all handover information at each stage of the patient's journey we have the potential to ensure that the patient's safety is paramount and optimal and timely care is delivered.

Further reading

Institute for Healthcare Improvement website: <http://www.ihi.org/ihi>
NHS Institute for Innovation and Improvement website: <http://www.institute.nhs.uk/>.
Scottish Patient Safety Programme website: <http://www.patientsafetyalliance.scot.nhs.uk>.

Conclusion

Part 2

Organ dysfunction

Heart

Left ventricular failure

The assessment and management of the LV is covered in other chapters of this book. The anatomy and physiology are summarized here, followed by reference to the relevant chapters covering functional assessment and management.

Anatomy and physiology of the LV

Anatomy

The LV receives oxygenated blood from the pulmonary veins and pumps it to the systemic circulation. It consists of:

- The mitral valve, forming the inlet to the ventricle
- The conical apical portion, containing fine trabeculations
- The outflow tract leading to the aortic valve.

The muscle fibres of the LV are formed in multiple overlapping sheets. Myocardial contractility is spiral, producing radial contractility and longitudinal shortening. The LV appears circular in short-axis view.

Physiology

- The systemic LV is a high-pressure system.
- Coronary perfusion occurs in diastole over four phases; isovolumic relaxation, rapid filling, diastasis, and atrial systole.
- Volume preloading increases stroke volume within the limits of the Starling effect.
- The ventricle responds to ↑ afterload through ↑ contractility and over time through muscle hypertrophy.

LV functional assessment

Cardiac output

Chapter 24 on central venous cannulation (CVC), pulmonary artery catheter (PAC) and minimally invasive CO monitoring describes the indications for and advantages of the invasive PAC and minimally invasive CO monitoring in the assessment and ongoing management of cardiogenic shock. The PAFC provides direct measurement of pulmonary pressures, SvO_2, and CO, while pulse contour analysis, thoracic bioimpedance measurement, and oesophageal Doppler provide minimally invasive derived measures of CO.

Anatomical and functional assessment

Chapter 32 on bedside echocardiography describes the indications of both transthoracic echocardiography (TTE) and transoesophageal echocardiography (TOE) in the CICU. The size, degree of filling, and contractility of the LV can be assessed. In addition, regional wall-motion abnormalities can be defined and culprit vessels identified.

Management of the failing LV

Management: general principles and the management of reversible causes

Chapter 7 on hypotension and low CO describes the general principles of managing patients with a poorly functioning LV following a standard ABC approach. In addition, identification and management of reversible causes including myocardial ischaemia are described.

Contractility: pharmacological support

Chapter 27 on circulatory support details the pharmacological actions of different classes of inotropes together with their indications. The selection and safe use of a particular vasoactive agent is based on knowledge of its cardiovascular effects, clinical indications, and an understanding of its clinical use.

Contractility: mechanical support

Chapter 27 on circulatory support goes on to describe the indications and use of mechanical and extracorporeal life support. This includes the use of IABP counterpulsation, short-term VADs, long-term VADs, and extracorporeal membrane oxygenation (ECMO).

Right ventricular failure

Anatomy and physiology of the RV

The RV differs from the LV in structure and function. The right side of the heart can be more difficult to assess and treat. Its interdependence with the LV highlights the importance of its careful assessment and optimization in the compromised patient.

Anatomy

The RV receives blood from systemic venous return and pumps it to the pulmonary circulation. It consists of:

- The sinus (inflow) below the tricuspid valve
- The free wall (providing contractility) which is thin walled
- The infundibulum (outflow) leading to the pulmonary valve.

The RV contracts in a peristaltic pattern from the sinus to the infundibulum. It relies on longitudinal shortening more than the LV.

The RV appears triangular when viewed from the side and crescentic when viewed in cross section.

Ventricular interdependence

The RV wraps around the LV: up to 30% of the contractile energy of the RV is generated by the LV.

The LV and RV are enclosed in a non-expanding pericardium. Overdistention of the RV within this closed sac compromises LV contractile performance primarily by reducing LV preload.

Physiology

- The RV is a low-pressure system (Fig. 11.1).
- RV wall stress is low. Coronary perfusion occurs in systole and diastole. An acute increase in afterload reduces coronary perfusion, so reducing contractile performance.
- Loss of forward flow from the RV increases RA pressure, reducing systemic venous return.

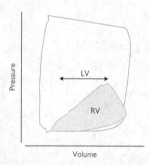

Figure 11.1 Pressure–volume loop. RV: ejection starts earlier in systole, and is against a low-resistance bed. Reproduced from *Heart*, F Sheehan and A Redington, 'Non-invasive imaging: the right ventricle: anatomy, physiology and clinical imaging', 94, 11, copyright 2008, with permission from BMJ Publishing Group Ltd.

The right ventricle

- Is a thin-walled low-pressure system.
- It is exquisitely volume sensitive.
- There is functional interdependence with the LV.
- The RVs response to ↑ preload or afterload is overdistention.

RV functional assessment

The complex morphology of the RV makes volume and functional assessment difficult. The current clinical standard is echocardiographic visual assessment of the RV with surrogate markers of contractility. Assessment should be corroborated in multiple views.

RV dilatation

TOE: mid-oesophageal four-chamber view or TTE: apical four-chamber view:

- RV should be approximately half LV size
- LV should form the apex.

Paradoxical septal motion

TOE: transgastric short-axis view of LV or TTE: parasternal short axis:

- Paradoxical septal motion in systole, reflecting the presence of RV systolic overload.

The patient in Fig. 11.2a exhibited normal septal motion with a pure spherical LV. The patient in Fig. 11.2b exhibited paradoxical septal motion at the end of systole and beginning of diastole reflecting systolic overload of the RV.

(a)   (b)

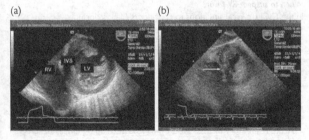

Figure 11.2 Short-axis view of the left ventricle by a transgastric approach. Reproduced from A. Vieillard-Baron, 'Assessment of right ventricular function', *Current Opinion in Critical Care*, 15, 3, pp. 254–260, copyright 2009, with permission from Wolters Kluwer.

Surrogate markers of contractility

TAPSE (normal > 16mm)

Tricuspid annular plane systolic excursion can be assessed in the TTE apical four-chamber view with M-mode, measuring the distance of tricuspid annular movement between end-diastole and end-systole.

Fractional area change (normal > 35%)

Other indirect measures of RV function include:

ECG
- RV strain
- New atrial fibrillation (AF).

Pulmonary artery floatation catheter
- The only way to directly measure right heart pressures. The gold standard for CO monitoring.
- Direct measurement of PAP allows continuous monitoring of therapy to reduce PAP.
- PAWP provides an indirect measure of left heart filling pressure and thus preload.

Management of the failing RV

RV function has often been overlooked in critically ill patients. The last decade has seen a significant advance in the understanding of RV haemodynamics and appreciation of their importance in global cardiac performance.

The RV can fail because of:
- Volume overload (*preload*)
- Impaired *contractility*, or
- Pressure overload (*afterload*).

When to suspect RV failure

In the CICU, clinical situations to consider RV failure include:
- Disproportionate rise in CVP (suggesting ↑ preload, particularly in association with tricuspid valve incompetence)
- Myocardial stunning following reperfusion
- RV ischaemia and infarction, either due to sustained hypotension or coronary occlusion
- When the LV is underfilled but the CVP is high and the RV is distended there may be RV failure
- Septic shock
- Pulmonary hypertension (primary or acquired)
- Acute respiratory distress syndrome (15% develop right heart failure)
- Secondary to LV failure (ventricular interdependence).

Management: general principles

Optimize ventilation
- FiO_2 to maintain normoxia
- Avoid high intrathoracic pressures:
  - Ventilate at 6–8mL/kg, avoid inspiratory pressure >30mmHg
  - Avoid auto-PEEP
- Avoid hypoxia, acidosis, and/or hypercarbia as these contribute to pulmonary vasoconstriction.

Maintain sinus rhythm (aim for HR 90–110bpm)
- Consider electrical cardioversion for atrial tachyarrhythmias
- Or pacing for symptomatic bradyarrhythmias.

Optimize preload
- If uncertain, 100mL crystalloid fluid challenge and assess response.
- If volume overloaded use IV diuretics in the first instance. If there is no response to diuretics consider ultrafiltration.
- If underfilled, decide on appropriate replacement fluid and continue to bolus in 100mL aliquots until euvolaemic.
- Support contractility:
  - Pharmacological (see ⬚ Pharmacological support, p. 288)
  - Surgical (see ⬚ Mechanical circulatory support: extracorporeal life support, p. 294).

Reduce afterload
- Pulmonary vasodilators such as inhaled nitric oxide, or nebulized iloprost.
- Once stable consider IV or oral vasodilators such as sildenafil or epoprostenol.
- Minimize blood production transfusion.

The general principles are described in Fig. 11.3.

Key point

In acute RV failure, every effort should be made to avoid systemic hypotension, which may lead to a vicious cycle of RV ischaemia and further hypotension.

Further reading

Haddad F, Couture P, Tousignant C, Denault AY. Right ventricular function in cardiovascular disease, part II: pathophysiology, clinical importance, and management of right ventricular failure. *Circulation* 2008;117:1717–31.

Contractility: pharmacological support

There is no evidence for the best inotrope regimen to use in right heart failure. Useful drugs are outlined here. Use should be tailored to the patient's haemodynamics and local guidelines. One logical sequence is suggested in the management algorithm (see Fig. 11.3).

Adrenaline
- *Infusion starting at 0.05mcg/kg/min (working range 0.02–0.2mcg/kg/min)*
- Useful resuscitation drug and first-line inotrope
- Direct acting on α_1, β_1, α_2 and β_2 receptors
- Undesirable effects:
  - Proarrhythmic
  - Hypertension
  - Hyperglycaemia
  - ↑ myocardial oxygen demand.

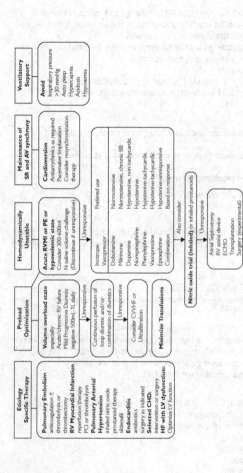

Figure 11.3 Management of acute RV failure. Haemodynamic instability is defined by hypotension or signs of low CO (e.g. renal failure). SR: sinus rhythm; PCI: percutaneous coronary intervention; AV: atrioventricular; ECMO: extracorporeal membrane oxygenation; CVVHF: continuous venovenous hemofiltration. Reproduced from F. Haddad, et al., 'Right ventricular function in cardiovascular disease, part II: pathophysiology, clinical importance, and management of right ventricular failure', *Circulation*, 117, 13, pp. 1717–1731, copyright 2008, with permission from American Heart Association and Wolters Kluwer.

Dopamine

- *Infusion starting at 5mcg/kg/min (working range 2.5–25mcg/kg/min)*
- Inotrope with vasoconstriction at higher concentrations
- Endogenous precursor of noradrenaline with predominantly β_1-receptor activity. At higher doses, inotropic effects mediated through β_1 receptors. Vasoconstrictor effects via α_1 and 5HT receptors.
- Undesirable effects:
  - Extravasation may cause local necrosis
  - Proarrhythmic secondary to abnormal calcium loading.

Milrinone

- *Infusion starting at 0.375mcg/kg/min (working range 0.1–0.75mcg/kg/min)*
- Inotrope and vasodilation
- Phosphodiesterase inhibitor inhibiting cAMP breakdown
- Undesirable effects:
  - Pro-arrhythmic
  - Often requires concomitant vasopressor.

Dobutamine

- *Infusion starting at 2.0mcg/kg/min (working range 0–20mcg/kg/min)*
- Inotrope, chronotrope, and vasodilator at higher doses
- Synthetic catecholamine acting on β_1, β_2, and α_1 receptors
- Undesirable effects:
  - Proarrhythmic
  - Hypotension at higher doses
  - Tachyphylaxis prolonged infusion over 96 hours has been associated with a decrease in the haemodynamic effect by as much as 50%.

Noradrenaline

- *Infusion starting at 0.05mcg/kg/min (working range 0.02–0.2mcg/kg/min)*
- Vasoconstriction
- Endogenous agonist at α_1 and α_2 adrenoreceptors (modest effect on β_1 adrenoreceptors)
- Undesirable effects:
  - Reduced renal and splanchnic blood flow
  - ↑ pulmonary vascular resistance (PVR)
  - Proarrhythmic.

Vasopressin

- *Infusion starting at 2IU/hour (working range 0–4IU/hour)*
- Direct vasoconstriction
- Peptide hormone agonist at AVPR1A receptor
- Undesirable effects:
  - Local tissue necrosis
  - Reduced splanchnic blood flow.

Phenylephrine

- *Infusion starting at 0.5mcg/kg/min (working range 0.4–9mcg/kg/min)*
- Vasopressor
- α_1 adrenoreceptors agonist

- Undesirable effects:
  - Arrhythmia including reflex bradycardia
  - Severe peripheral and visceral vasoconstriction.

Mechanical support

Mechanical cardiac support for short-term use covers a spectrum of techniques that can be classified as follows:
- Intra-aortic counter pulsation with an IABP
- Extracorporeal ventricular support—*short-term*:
  - Short-term VADs
  - ECMO.

In patients with severe RV dysfunction, a right ventricular assist device (RVAD) may be considered. RVADs may be used alone or in combination with LVADs.

Short-term VADs have a potential duration of support of days to weeks. An exit strategy must be identified before device implantation. This may be ventricular recovery, or as bridge to destination therapy or transplantation. If there is associated hypoxia there may be benefit in combining short-term ventricular support with oxygenation in an ECMO circuit.

Commonly used short-term devices in the UK include the Levitronix CentriMag™ VAD. This device can act as a RVAD, LVAD, or BiVAD. The pump is outside the body. Flow is non-pulsatile, but residual ventricular ejection may add pulsatility.

See 🕮 Mechanical circulatory support: extracorporeal life support, p. 294 for further discussion of mechanical circulatory support.

Key point

An exit strategy should always be identified before embarking on any form of mechanical support.

Further reading

Shuhaiber JH, Jenkins D, Berman M, Parameshwar J, Dhital K, Tsui S, et al. The Papworth experience with the Levitronix CentriMag ventricular assist device. *J Heart Lung Transplant* 2008;27:158–64.

Afterload reduction

Pulmonary hypertension

- Mean pulmonary artery pressure ≥25mmHg at rest or >30mmHg on exercise.

Acute management options in severe pulmonary hypertension:
- Seek expert help.
- High-flow oxygen is a potent pulmonary vasodilator.
- Specific pulmonary vasodilator therapy—first line:
  - If intubated, inhaled nitric oxide
  - If not intubated, nebulized iloprost.
- IV and oral agents may be used to wean inhaled nitric oxide, consider sildenafil, epoprostenol.
- Consider ECMO ± RVAD if the RV is failing despite medical therapy.

- Atrial septostomy is used in chronic pulmonary hypertension, but may be considered in the acute setting. This creates a right-to-left shunt at atrial level with afterload reduction of the right heart. This is at the expense of resultant cyanosis.

Nitric oxide
- *Delivered via a dedicated ventilator circuit*
- *Start at 20ppm (range 0–20ppm)*
- Smooth muscle relaxation mediated through cGMP
- Undesirable effects:
  - Humidification should be avoided to prevent formation of nitric acid
  - Withdrawal should be cautious to avoid rebound pulmonary hypertension.

Iloprost
- *First dose: 2.5mcg nebulized*
- *Thereafter: 5mcg 6–9 times/day (>2 hours apart)*
- Inhaled prostacyclin PGI$_2$
- Undesirable effects:
  - Systemic hypotension.

Sildenafil
- *IV 10mg three times a day (named patient prescription)*
- *Oral 20mg three times a day*
- Phosphodiesterase-5 inhibitor, blocks metabolism of nitric oxide
- Undesirable effects:
  - Systemic hypotension and headache.

Epoprostenol (Flolan®)
- *Infusion starting at 2ng/kg/min*
- *Increment by 1–2ng/kg/min every 15 minutes*
- Prostacyclin
- Short half-life, potential to titrate in the unstable patient
- Undesirable effects:
  - *Avoid in severe LVSD*
  - Hypotension
  - Flushing, headache.

Reversible causes
Reversible causes should be identified and treated once initial management is underway.

RV myocardial stunning
- Transient (usually up to 24 hours) systolic and diastolic dysfunction persisting after ischaemia and subsequent reperfusion.
- Intraoperative volatile anaesthesia offers pre-conditioning benefit.
- Inotropic support improves performance of stunned myocardium.

RV myocardial infarction
- Classical triad of hypotension, elevated CVP, and clear lung fields.
- Diagnosis:

- ECG: ST elevation in inferior (II, III, and aVF) and/or right ventricular leads (right-sided chest leads). Caution not to overlook posterior changes (ST *depression* in V1–3 with dominant R-wave pattern).
- Echo: this is the key diagnostic tool demonstrating that the RV is dilated with systolic dysfunction.
- If this occurs in the postoperative period after cardiac surgery immediate revascularization should be considered. This may be surgical but is increasingly achieved with PCI. Time is myocardium!

Pulmonary hypertension—acquired, mitral valve disease

- Severe mitral stenosis (valve area <1.0cm^2) is associated with reversible pulmonary hypertension. Supportive measures may be required in the immediate postoperative phase after mitral valve replacement.
- Untreated severe mitral stenosis can be diagnosed with echocardiography. TOE will demonstrate the mechanism of the valve lesion and can identify whether transcatheter balloon valvuloplasty is feasible. If not then urgent valve surgery may be required.

Pulmonary hypertension—acquired, thromboembolic disease

- Although rare in the immediate postoperative period in cardiac surgery, pulmonary embolism (PE) may be seen in long-term patients and those admitted for non-surgical care.
- PE presenting with cardiogenic shock has a mortality of 20–50%.
- Management of acute PE depends on the severity of haemodynamic consequence. If there are no features of shock (tachycardia or hypotension) then anticoagulation with heparin is sufficient. If the patient is haemodynamically compromised by PE then the clot should be dispersed. The options include:
  - Thrombolysis
  - Catheter fragmentation
  - Surgical embolectomy.

Valve heart disease

Aortic stenosis

Aetiology

The majority of patients with symptomatic aortic stenosis (AS) are elderly. The predominant aetiology is degenerative calcific valve disease. Some may present because of rheumatic heart disease and may have other valve involvement.

In a young person there should be a high index of suspicion of a congenitally abnormal valve, e.g. bicuspid. This has an association with aortic coarctation.

The differential diagnosis for AS is LVOT obstruction.

Definition

- Transvalvular velocity and hence gradient is dependent on LV systolic function, and should be interpreted in this context. A patient with poor LV function will generate a lower gradient across a valve with reduced area than a patient with a good ventricle. See Table 11.1.
- Timing of corrective intervention is determined by the presence or absence of symptoms.

Table 11.1 Quantification of aortic stenosis

	Valve area	Mean gradient	Jet velocity
Mild	>1.5cm^2	<25mmHg	<3.0m/s
Moderate	1.0–1.5cm^2	25–40mmHg	3.0–4.0m/s
Severe	<1.0cm^2	>40mmHg	>4.0m/s

Pathophysiology

The LV undergoes concentric hypertrophy to overcome LV outflow obstruction. The ↑ wall tension together with thickened myocardium renders the endocardium vulnerable to ischaemia. The ventricle may then progress to fail. The failing ventricle will dilate and the walls will progressively thin.

Natural history

There is a long latent period in the development of AS where patients remain asymptomatic and the risk of sudden death is low. The presentation of severe AS is with dyspnoea, exercise limitation, and syncope. The average survival after the onset of symptoms is 2–3 years with a high risk of sudden death.

Management options

Surgical aortic valve replacement (AVR) is indicated in patients with:
- Symptomatic severe AS
- Severe or moderate AS when undergoing surgery to the coronaries, the aorta or other heart valves.

Surgical AVR may be considered in patients with asymptomatic AS when:
- There is an abnormal response to exercise or a likelihood of rapid progression of disease. In addition if valve area is <0.6cm^2 and predicted surgical mortality is low
- LV systolic dysfunction.

Percutaneous aortic balloon valvuloplasty may be considered:
- In a haemodynamically unstable adult as a bridge to surgery
- As palliation in a patient with severe AS who is unfit for surgery.

Transcatheter aortic valve implantation is an alternative to AVR in patients:
- At high risk because of comorbidities
- With a hostile chest—previous sternotomy, thoracic radiotherapy, porcelain aorta precluding aortic cannulation.

Postoperative pitfalls

While the postoperative course of the patient undergoing AVR follows the typical pattern outlined in Part 1 of this book, there are unique pitfalls to be aware of:
- The hypertrophied LV is at risk of poor myocardial protection, and so may have a prolonged period of stunning after CPB.
- The stunned heart is volume sensitive and requires careful attention to maintaining preload. There is a dependence on atrial filling, and DDD pacing is preferred. In addition, the hypertrophied myocardium requires a high perfusion pressure to maintain endocardial perfusion and may require vasopressors.
- Typically, once contractile function has returned, the ventricle is contracting against a reduced afterload, and so there is a tendency to systemic hypertension.
- AV dissociation is a recognized postoperative complication and a proportion of patients will require permanent pacing.
- All patients will require attention to postoperative anticoagulation.

Subaortic obstruction

Subaortic stenosis may present as a fixed or dynamic obstruction below the level of the aortic valve. It may present *de novo* or consequent to mitral valve (MV) repair or AV surgery.

Aetiology

- Hypertrophic obstructive cardiomyopathy (HOCM) is morphologically characterized by LV hypertrophy, and may have associated MV anomaly. Subaortic obstruction occurs in the form with high septal hypertrophy or a sigmoid septum.
- Systolic anterior motion (SAM) of the anterior leaflet of the MV may occur after MV repair when the anterior leaflet of the MV is sucked into the LVOT by the Venturi effect.
- Mid-ventricular obstruction and SAM after aortic surgery.
- Fixed discrete subaortic stenosis, which may occur in association with other congenital anomalies (VSD, patent ductus arteriosus, coarctation of aorta), or may be an acquired lesion.

Presentation

Presentation may range from mild exertional symptoms to syncope and in the surgical patient as failure to wean from CPB.

Management

Medical management focuses on:
- Maintenance of sinus rhythm with a slow normal HR
- Avoid hypovolaemia
- Avoid the use of inotropes.

Surgical correction of the underlying lesion provides definitive treatment.

Aortic regurgitation—chronic

Aetiology

Chronic aortic regurgitation (AR) most commonly presents in the elderly as a degenerative disease.

Definition

Chronic AR is always associated with ↑ LV dimensions. The timing of corrective intervention is determined by LV function *and dimensions*. See Table 11.2.

Table 11.2 Quantification of chronic aortic regurgitation

	Colour Doppler jet width of LVOT	Doppler vena contracta width	Regurgitant fraction
Mild	<25% LVOT	<0.3cm	<30%
Moderate		0.3–0.6cm	30–50%
Severe	>65%LVOT	>0.6cm	>50%

Pathophysiology

The LV is volume overloaded. There is an increase in end-diastolic volume. ↑ compliance prevents an increase in end-diastolic pressure and the ventricle hypertrophies to maintain EF. Over time the end-diastolic pressure increases, the LV dilates, and the thickened myocardium renders the endocardium vulnerable to ischaemia. The ventricle may then progress to fail.

Natural history

There is a long latent period in the progression of disease. Prognosis is associated with LV size rather than onset of symptoms. Regular follow-up and imaging is thus essential.

Management options
- Surgical AVR is indicated in patients with:
  - Severe AR who are symptomatic or have LV systolic dysfunction
  - Severe AR who are undergoing CABG
- Surgical AVR is reasonable in patients with:
  - Severe AR, preserved LV systolic function, but severely dilated LV (>75mm)
- Surgical AVR may be considered in patients with:
  - Moderate AR who are undergoing surgery on the ascending aorta or coronary arteries.

Postoperative pitfalls

The LV is dilated, may have reduced systolic function, and is working against an ↑ afterload following valve replacement:

- The ventricle will require careful attention to maintain pre-load.
- Consider early institution of inotropic support.
- AV dissociation is a recognized postoperative complication and a proportion of patients will require permanent pacing.
- All patients will require attention to postoperative anticoagulation.

Aortic regurgitation—acute

Aetiology

Acute AR is most commonly associated with bacterial endocarditis and aortic dissection. Typically the LV is not dilated.

Definition

Classification of severity is the same as in chronic AR but the LV dimensions are unchanged. See Table 11.3.

Table 11.3 Quantification of acute aortic regurgitation

	Colour Doppler jet width of LVOT	Doppler vena contracta width	Regurgitant fraction
Mild	<25% LVOT	<0.3cm	<30%
Moderate		0.3–0.6cm	30–50%
Severe	>65% LVOT	>0.6cm	>50%

Pathophysiology

The acute volume loading of the non-adapted LV results in ↑ LV end-diastolic and left atrial pressures. Patients typically present in pulmonary oedema and cardiogenic shock. This deterioration is exacerbated in patients with a poorly compliant ventricle, for example, the hypertensive patient who presents with AR secondary to aortic dissection.

Natural history

Death due to pulmonary oedema, ventricular arrhythmias, electromechanical dissociation, or circulatory collapse is common in acute severe AR, even with intensive medical management. The timing of surgical intervention in patients with bacterial endocarditis depends on the degree of compromise. Ideally the infection is eradicated at the time of surgery by 6 weeks of antibiotics. Sometimes the patient's deteriorating clinical condition precludes this.

Management options

The timing of surgical intervention in patients with bacterial endocarditis depends on the degree of cardiorespiratory compromise. Ideally a full course of antibiotics will be completed preoperatively.

Medical management may temporize clinical deterioration:

- Dobutamine or dopamine to augment forward flow and GTN to reduce after load
- AVR provides definitive treatment.

Postoperative pitfalls
As for patients after AVR for AR, with the compounding variable of a septic picture.

Aortic regurgitation—functional

Aetiology
Functional AR is caused by aortic root dilatation. The valve is usually morphologically normal with a dilated annulus. Typically the LV is not dilated.

Definition
Classification of severity is the same as in chronic AR. LV dimensions are unchanged.

Pathophysiology
The pathophysiology of functional AR mirrors chronic AR. Volume overloading of the LV leads to progressive dilation and eventual decompensation of the ventricle.

Management options
Decision-making considers both the sequele of the AR and the disease of the ascending aorta.

The aortic root may be abnormal because of Marfan's syndrome, dissection, or chronic dilatation secondary to hypertension or a bicuspid aortic valve.

In general, AVR and aortic root reconstruction are indicated in patients with disease of the aortic root or proximal aorta and AR of any severity when:
- Dilatation of the aorta or aortic root reaches or exceeds 5.0cm by echocardiography (some consider surgery at 4.5cm)
- Based on a rate of increase of 0.5cm per year or greater.

Postoperative pitfalls
The postoperative management is as for patients after AVR for AR, with the additional caveat that the systolic pressure should be controlled to protect the ascending aorta.

Mitral stenosis

Aetiology
Mitral stenosis (MS) is most commonly secondary to rheumatic carditis.

Congenital MS is rare as are other acquired causes of MV obstruction. Other causes include left atrial myxoma, ball valve thrombus, mucopolysaccharidosis, and severe annular calcification.

Definition
Mitral stenosis is an obstruction to LV inflow at the level of the mitral valve. Normal MV area is 4–5cm^2. See Table 11.4.

Table 11.4 Quantification of mitral stenosis

	Valve area	Pressure half time	Mean pressure drop
Mild	1.6–2.0cm^2	71–139ms	<5mmHg
Moderate	1.0–1.5cm^2	140–219ms	5–10mmHg
Severe	<1.0cm^2	>219ms	>10mmHg

Pathophysiology

There is progressive dilation of the LA, with subsequent development of AF, pulmonary hypertension and the risk of atrial clot formation which may embolize systemically.

Natural history

Patients remain asymptomatic while the MV area is >1.5cm^2. Symptoms of dyspnoea are associated with reduced cardiac output and ↑ flow across the MV, initially with exercise and subsequently at rest. Symptoms accelerate with the development of atrial arrhythmias and pulmonary hypertension.

Management options

MV surgery is indicated for patients with severe MS and moderate MS associated with severe symptoms, pulmonary hypertension, or coexisting moderate to severe MR.

Postoperative pitfalls

While the postoperative course of the patient undergoing MVR follows the typical pattern outlined in Part 1 of this book, there are unique pitfalls to be aware of:

- Pulmonary hypertension may take months to resolve after MVR and patients are prone to right heart failure in the immediate postoperative phase.
- AF is common postoperatively.

Mitral regurgitation—organic

Aetiology

Organic MR incudes all aetiologies where leaflet abnormalities are the cause of the regurgitation. There is a declining incidence of rheumatic fever and degenerative changes are now the most common cause of organic MR.

Definition

See Table 11.5.

Table 11.5 Quantification of organic mitral regurgitation

	Vena contracta	Jet area/LA	PISA radius
Mild	<0.3cm	<20%	<0.4cm
Moderate	0.3–0.7cm	21–39%	0.4–1.0cm
Severe	>0.7cm	>40%	>1.0cm

Pathophysiology

There is progressive dilation of the LV with deterioration of LV systolic function as the end-diastolic dimension (EDD) increases. Caution in interpreting LV systolic function must be exercised, as the MR can flatter the appearance of the ventricular function.

At the same time the LA is volume overloaded and AF and pulmonary hypertension secondary to pulmonary congestion may develop.

Natural history

MR may develop acutely, and patients present with rapidly developing symptoms or it may develop chronically with symptoms of more insidious onset.

Patients develop symptoms of LV failure as the function of the LV deteriorates, or when they decompensate with AF. The development of pulmonary hypertension is associated with breathlessness.

Management options

The mitral valve may be surgically repaired or replaced. When replaced the mitral valve apparatus may be preserved or removed.

While there are no randomized trials it is accepted that where feasible and the expertise exists, mitral valve repair is the optimal surgical treatment. Preservation of the MV apparatus leads to better postoperative LV function.

Surgery is indicated in acute severe MR. Patients with chronic MR are considered for surgery when they become symptomatic, and develop AF or pulmonary hypertension.

Postoperative pitfalls

The management of the postoperative patient follows the pattern outlined in Part 1 of this book:

- The LV tends to have a high EDD and requires careful attention to preload.
- Pulmonary hypertension may take months to resolve and patients may be prone to right heart failure in the immediate postoperative period.

Mitral valve prolapse

Definition

Mitral valve prolapse (MVP) is the systolic billowing of one or both mitral leaflets into the LA. It may or may not be associated with MR.

By definition, the valve prolapse is of 2mm or more above the mitral annulus in the long-axis parasternal view and other views.

Aetiology

MV prolapse can be familial or non-familial.

Natural history

The natural history of MVP is heterogeneous with most following a benign course.

When associated with MR, MVP will progress to dilatation of the LA and subsequent development of AF and pulmonary hypertension secondary to venous congestion. MR may also result in LV dysfunction and congestive heart failure.

If a chordae ruptures, the mitral valve leaflet may become flail.

Management options and postoperative pitfalls
As for mitral regurgitation—organic.

Mitral regurgitation—functional

Aetiology
The mitral valve is structurally normal and the MR results from changes in LV geometry secondary to ischaemic changes. Functional MR is seen in LV dysfunction of ischaemic origin and cardiomyopathy.

Natural history
Functional MR is associated with a poorer prognosis, as by definition it is associated with LV dysfunction.

Management options
The evidence base for the management of functional MR is weak. The predominant surgical technique is restrictive annuloplasty ring at the time of coronary revascularization when the MR is severe. Historically the operative risk is perceived as high; however, case series from experienced centres give good results. The management of mild or moderate MR is less clear.

Postoperative pitfalls
As for mitral regurgitation—organic.

Tricuspid valve regurgitation

Definition
Trivial tricuspid regurgitation (TR) is frequently seen on echocardiography. Pathological TR is usually associated with RV dysfunction secondary to volume or pressure overload. See Table 11.6.

Table 11.6 Quantification of tricuspid valve regurgitation

	Hepatic vein flow	Vena contracta	Jet area/LA	PISA radius
Mild	Sys dominance	Undefined	<5cm^2	<0.5cm
Mod	Sys blunting	<0.7cm	5–10cm^2	0.6–0.9cm
Severe	Sys reversal	>0.7cm	>10cm^2	>0.9cm

Aetiology and pathophysiology
Severe TR is nearly always consequent to annular dilatation and RV dysfunction, whether it be because of pressure or volume overload.
- RV pressure overload:
  - Left-sided heart disease
  - Cor pulmonale
  - Idiopathic pulmonary hypertension
- RV volume overload:
  - Atrial septal defects
  - Intrinsic RV disease
- Primary TR may result from trauma or endocarditis.

Natural history

Severe TR may be well tolerated for years, but ultimately has a high mortality. Operative intervention is associated with high mortality and the challenge of managing patients with severe TR is the decision-making regarding timing of surgery.

Management options

The predominant surgical technique is the insertion of an annuloplasty ring. Valve replacement carries an operative mortality of 7–40%.

Postoperative pitfalls

The management of the postoperative patient follows the pattern outlined in Part 1 of this book.

In addition this group of patients is particularly vulnerable to right heart failure. See 📖 Management of the failing RV, p. 88.

Tricuspid valve stenosis

Aetiology

Tricuspid stenosis (TS) is uncommon but may be seen with rheumatic carditis. It may be missed, as commonly the MV symptoms predominate.

Right atrial masses may present a non-valvular obstruction of the RV.

Definition

TS is an obstruction to RV inflow at the level of the tricuspid valve. Normal TV area is >7.0cm^2. See Table 11.7.

Table 11.7 Quantification of tricuspid valve stenosis

	Valve area	Mean pressure drop	Inflow VTI
Normal	>7.0cm^2	–	
Severe	<1.0cm^2	>5mmHg	>60cm

Pathophysiology and natural history

The presentation of TS is usually over shadowed by associated valve abnormalities.

Signs of progressive right heart failure may develop.

Management options

TV balloon valvuloplasty may be considered, but is associated with a high incidence of subsequent TR.

Conservative surgery or valve replacement dependent on the presenting anatomy and local expertise.

Postoperative pitfalls

While the postoperative course of the patient undergoing TV replacement follows the typical pattern outlined in Part 1 of this book, patients are vulnerable to right heart failure. See 📖 Management of the failing RV, p. 88.

Pulmonary valve

Disorder of the pulmonary valve is usually associated with congenital heart disorders. For discussion regarding the pulmonary valve, see Chapter 19 on adult patients with congenital heart disease.

Common arrhythmias and their management

Bradyarrhythmias

Postoperative bradyarrhythmias requiring permanent pacemaker implantation occur in up to 4% of patients, most commonly after aortic valve surgery. The most common abnormalities are a nodal rhythm, sinus node dysfunction, and complete AV block. A further group of patients require heart rate support in the immediate postoperative period to achieve a target heart rate.

Epicardial pacing is the mainstay of heart rate in the postoperative phase. Transvenous pacing provides the backstop. Transcutaneous pacing and pharmacological therapies are useful to temporize.

Pacing

Most postoperative patients have epicardial pacing leads and their heart rates can be controlled (see 📖 Introduction, p. 304).

Transcutaneous pacing may be administered through an external defibrillator as a temporizing measure when the bradyarrhythmia is associated with a low BP and no other therapy is immediately available. Heart rate is selected and gain ↑ until capture is achieved. It is uncomfortable for the patient, who may require sedation.

Transvenous pacing requires the placement of a transvenous temporary pacing wire in the RV under X-ray guidance.

Pharmacological management

Atropine

- Bolus 0.1–0.6 mg
- Max. 3mg
- Anticholinergic, increases firing at SA node increasing heart rate
- Competitive antagonist for muscarinic acetyl-choline receptor, reducing parasympathetic activity
- Undesirable effects:
  - Short-acting and ineffective in AV block
  - Vasodilation
  - Reduced sweating and lacrimation
  - Central nervous system (CNS) effects—confusion, excitation
  - Dilated pupils.

Isoprenaline

- Bolus 20mcg
- Then infusion 1–4mcg/min titrated to response
- Sympathomimetic β1and β2 adrenergic agonist
- Chronotrope, ionotrope, and peripheral vasodilation effects
- Undesirable effects:
  - Proarrhythmic
  - Rarely paradoxical airways resistance requiring cessation of the drug.

Consider both directly and indirectly acting chronotropes, e.g. adrenaline (direct) and dobutamine (indirect) if both inotropy and chronotropy is appropriate to the patient's condition.

Tachyarrhythmias—atrial fibrillation

Tachyarrhythmias, particularly AF occur in up to 40% of patients following CABG and in up to 60% of patients following CABG and valve replacement.

Risk

The risk of postoperative AF is highest in those with preoperative AF, ↑ age, impaired LVEF, and hypokalaemia and hypomagnesaemia. Peak incidence is on day 3.

Prophylaxis

There is some evidence for pharmacological prophylaxis of AF. The maintenance of potassium, magnesium, and calcium within the high normal range is effective first-line prophylaxis.

Amiodarone and β-blockers may be considered for prophylaxis of AF following cardiac surgery.

Treatment

Patients in AF with haemodynamic compromise should have synchronized DC cardioversion.

Rate control

AF without haemodynamic compromise following CABG can be treated with rate limiting therapy as 80% revert to sinus rhythm spontaneously within 24 hours and 90% revert spontaneously within 6 weeks.

Treatment options for rate limitation include the following:
- Electrolytes: the maintenance of potassium, magnesium, and calcium within the high normal range.
- Amiodarone provides rate control with the additional benefit that the patient may chemically cardiovert.
- β-blockers provide good rate control, but are not always appropriate to start in the very early postoperative period.
- Digoxin may be considered for rate control in AF.

Persisting AF

AF is more likely to persist following valve surgery and may persist in a small number of patients following CABG.

Anticoagulation for patients with AF persisting for 48 hours should be considered on a case-by-case basis. The benefit of preventing thrombotic emboli and stroke needs to be weighed against the risk of bleeding in the postoperative period.

Patients who tolerate rate-controlled AF may not require cardioversion. Those who tolerate it poorly should be considered for chemical cardioversion or for elective synchronized DC cardioversion.

Where pharmacological therapy is used to treat AF, the need for persisting therapy should be reviewed within 6 weeks of hospital discharge.

Tachyarrhythmias—ventricular

Ventricular tachycardias associated with CABG have a variable effect on prognosis. Non-sustained VT and VF is commonly seen when coming off bypass, it is thought to be re-perfusion induced, and is typically benign. Ventricular tachycardias occurring later in the clinical course may be associated with a reversible underlying pathology such as cardiac tamponade or myocardial ischaemia which should be identified and treated.

Prophylaxis

- Amiodarone is indicated for prophylaxis against ventricular arrhythmias in cardiac surgery.
- Maintenance of electrolytes (potassium, magnesium, and calcium) in the high normal range is indicated for prophylaxis against ventricular arrhythmias in cardiac surgery.

Pulseless VF and VT; VT with a pulse and haemodynamic compromise

Patients with VF or pulseless VT should be defibrillated immediately.

Those with VT and a pulse who have haemodynamic compromise may require sedation before cardioversion.

Patients with refractory VF or pulseless VT should be managed by the CALS algorithm with early sternal re-opening, internal cardiac massage, and internal defibrillation. They may require re-institution of cardio-pulmonary bypass (see ▢ Cardiac Surgery Advanced Life Support, p. 26).

VT with a pulse and no haemodynamic compromise

Even in the absence of haemodynamic compromise, patients with persistent VT require cardioversion. This may be pharmacological with amiodarone, or electrical with synchronized DC cardioversion. Patients who are conscious will require sedation for this.

Special circumstance

Torsade de point (polymorphic VT characterized by a change in amplitude of the QRS complexes with twisting around an isoelectric line) in an otherwise stable patient is managed medically with magnesium.

Further reading

Scottish Intercollegiate Guidelines Network (SIGN). *Cardiac Arrhythmias in Coronary Heart Disease.* SIGN Guideline 94. Edinburgh: SIGN; 2007.

Lung

Acute lung injury/acute respiratory distress syndrome

Introduction

Acute respiratory distress syndrome (ARDS) is a clinical condition comprising respiratory distress, hypoxaemia refractory to oxygen, ↓ lung compliance, and the appearance of diffuse infiltrates on a CXR.

Definition

ARDS is the severe form of a disease spectrum that occurs in the lungs of critically ill patients. Acute lung injury (ALI) is the 'milder' form of the spectrum and although it has a similar pathogenesis, it has a better outcome.

The diagnostic criteria for ALI/ARDS are as follows:
- The onset is acute
- The presence of bilateral pulmonary infiltrates on a CXR
- The pulmonary artery wedge pressure (PAWP) is ≤18mmHg or no clinical evidence of left atrial hypertension
- In ALI the PaO_2/FiO_2 ratio is <40 (300mmHg)
- In ARDS the PaO_2/FiO_2 ratio is <27 (200mmHg).

The Murray Lung Injury Score can stratify severe acute respiratory failure (Table 12.1).

Table 12.1 The Murray Lung Injury Score

Score	0	1	2	3	4
PaO_2/FiO_2 (mmHg)	≥300	225–299	175–224	100–174	<100
Chest radiographic alveolar consolidation	None	1 quadrant	2 quadrants	3 quadrants	4 quadrants
PEEP (cmH_2O)	≤5	6–8	9–11	12–14	≥15
Compliance	≥80	60–79	40–59	20–39	≤19

The final value is obtained by dividing the aggregate sum by the number of components that were used.

No lung injury	0
Mild–moderate lung injury	0.1–2.5
Severe lung injury	>2.5

Reprinted with permission of the American Thoracic Society. Copyright © 2014 American Thoracic Society. Murray JF Matthay MA et al. An expanded definition of the adult respiratory distress syndrome. *Am Rev Respir Dis.* 1988; 138: 720–723. Official Journal of the American Thoracic Society.

Incidence

The reported incidence of ALI varies widely; incidence ranging from 16–34 per 100,000 person-years in Europe and Australia whereas in the US the incidence is 78 per 100,000 person-years.

Two decades ago the mortality ranged from 50–70% but has since declined and is now in the region of 30–40%. This is similar in patients who present with ALI or ARDS. The cause for the decline is not entirely clear but advances in general supportive care and the use of ventilatory strategies may account for the change.

Risk factors

There is a probable genetic predisposition with higher death rates in African Americans and males:

- Pulmonary risk factors:
  - Pneumonia
  - Aspiration
  - Lung contusion
  - Inhalational injury
  - PE
  - Drowning
- Extrapulmonary risk factors:
  - Sepsis
  - Shock
  - Trauma
  - Pancreatitis
  - Blood transfusion
  - CPB.

In recent years transfusion-related ALI (TRALI) and novel viral pathogens (severe acute respiratory syndrome or SARS) have emerged as important risk factors for the development of ALI.

Pathophysiology

The acute phase

- Disruption of the normal alveolar–capillary barrier allowing protein-rich fluid to leak into alveoli; neutrophils, red blood cells, and fibroblasts all enter alveoli.
- Pro-inflammatory cytokines are secreted by alveolar macrophages.
- Anti-inflammatory cytokines are also found in the alveoli, but in ALI/ARDS the balance is disrupted and the pro-inflammatory effect predominates.
- Other mechanisms in the acute phase involve coagulation abnormalities leading to microvascular occlusion in the lungs due to platelet and fibrin-rich thrombi and abnormal fibrinolysis.

The resolution phase

- Depends on repair of the alveolar epithelium and removal of the protein-rich fluid from the alveolar space.
- Proliferation of type II cells occurs which then differentiate into type I cells.
- Removal of alveolar fluid dependent on active transport of sodium via type II cells, and then water follows by osmosis via channels on type I cells.
- Insoluble proteins removed by macrophages and neutrophil clearance may be by apoptosis.

Fibrosing alveolitis
- Associated with a higher mortality.
- May begin as early as 5–7 days after onset of ALI/ARDS.
- Alveolar spaces get filled with inflammatory cells, fibrin, collagen, and blood vessels leading to fibrosis.

Management

The management of ALI/ARDS is aimed at:
- Identifying and treating the underlying cause:
  - Consider antimicrobial therapy
  - Consider surgical drainage of an intra-abdominal collection
  - Removal of invasive lines in the case of a catheter-related blood stream infection
- Providing supportive care:
  - Adequate nutrition
  - Stress ulcer prophylaxis
  - DVT prophylaxis
  - Haemodynamic management
  - Optimal fluid management remains unclear. Conservative strategy associated with improved lung function and ↓ duration of mechanical ventilation and intensive care
- Maintaining oxygenation using a protective ventilatory strategy. Ventilating at high tidal volumes (volutrauma) and pressures (barotrauma) can cause disruption of the alveolar–capillary interface; biotrauma (the release of inflammatory cytokines from neutrophils) is due to shearing forces as collapsed alveoli are repeatedly opened and closed and can lead to distant organ damage:
  - The ARDSnet group have published a table looking at the combinations of FiO_2 and PEEP for maintaining arterial oxygenation in ARDS (Table 12.2)
- Achieving PaO_2 >8kPa or SpO_2 88–95%.

Lung-protective strategies

- FiO_2: accept a PaO_2 >8kPa. Prolonged high concentrations of oxygen can contribute to lung injury due to oxygen toxicity
- *PEEP* (positive end-expiratory pressure) improves oxygenation by recruiting collapsed alveoli, improving ventilation/perfusion (V/Q) matching, and reducing intrapulmonary shunt.
- *Low tidal volume ventilation:*
  - Maintain a tidal volume of 6mL/kg using predicted body weight
  - Keep the peak airway pressure <30cmH$_2$O
  - Permissive hypercapnia (pH >7.1).

Table 12.2 The ARDSnet group combinations of FiO_2 and PEEP for maintaining arterial oxygenation in ARDS

FiO_2	PEEP (cm H_2O)
0.3	5
0.4	5–8
0.5	8–10
0.6	10
0.7	10–14
0.8	14
0.9	16–18
1.0	18–24

Data from The Acute Respiratory Distress Syndrome Network, 'Ventilation with lower tidal volumes as compared with traditional tidal volumes for acute lung injury and the acute respiratory distress syndrome', *The New England Journal of Medicine*, 342, 18, pp. 1301–1308.

Alternative strategies for improving profound hypoxaemia include:

- *Recruitment manoeuvres (RM) and high PEEP*:
  - The aim is to open up previously collapsed and flooded alveoli which should lead to improved oxygenation and a reduction in ventilator-induced lung injury from the shear stresses from repetitive opening and closing of alveoli.
  - However, 'normal' alveoli will be subjected to the risk of overdistension and damage and there is a possibility of haemodynamic compromise.
  - RM with high PEEP or high PEEP alone is best considered early in ARDS with severe hypoxaemia when plateau airway pressures are <30cmH$_2$O.
  - Do not consider these strategies in patients with pneumothoraces or when the disease is focal.
- *Prone positioning*:
  - V/Q mismatch is improved by recruiting dependent atelectatic lung areas.
  - Oxygenation does improve, but there is no clear evidence that mortality is reduced.
  - There are technical difficulties associated with turning patients, such as accidental dislodgement of invasive catheters and endotracheal/tracheostomy tubes as well as the risk of pressure ulcers and facial oedema.
- *High-frequency oscillatory ventilation (HFOV)*:
  - Uses high airway pressure to achieve lung recruitment and thus improve oxygenation.
  - An oscillating piston creates cycles of pressure above and below the mean airway pressure at a high frequency with small tidal volumes.
  - Should not be used in patients with shock, airway obstruction, intracranial haemorrhage, or refractory barotrauma.
  - Sedation is needed and severe acidosis may occur due to limited CO_2 excretion.

- *Inhaled nitric oxide:*
  - A potent vasodilator which promotes the distribution of blood flow towards ventilated portions of the lung minimizing V/Q mismatch and improving oxygenation.
  - Little systemic absorption and rapidly inactivated.
- *Steroids:*
  - Steroids could stop the progression to severe ALI/ARDS by inhibiting neutrophil activation, collagen deposition, and the proliferation of fibroblasts.
  - Clinical trials have failed to show a benefit to patients given steroids in early ALI and an ↑ mortality was noted in patients given steroids after 14 days of diagnosis.
  - Routine use is not to be recommended but could be considered in life-threatening hypoxaemia when other measures have failed.
  - Low dose of methylprednisolone (1mg/kg/day) should be used, and stopped if no improvement occurs after 3 days.
- *Extracorporeal lung support (ECLS):*
  - Veno-venous life support circuit that removes blood from the patient and circulates it through a membrane oxygenator providing gaseous exchange and allowing the lungs to recover. There are two main types of ECLS that have been used: extracorporeal membrane oxygenation (ECMO) which is a modified form of cardiopulmonary bypass and extracorporeal CO_2 removal.
  - The main risks are due to the need for anticoagulation and large-bore central venous cannulae. The CESAR trial (Conventional ventilation or ECMO for severe adult respiratory failure) showed an improvement in the survival and absence of severe disability at 6 months in the intervention group.
  - ECMO or extracorporeal CO_2 removal should only be considered when all other therapies have failed and at a centre with experience in extracorporeal lung support. It should not be used in patients with contraindications to anticoagulation and in those patients ventilated with high airway pressures for >7 days.

Further reading

ARDS Clinical Network website: ℛ <http://www.ardsnet.org>.

Ventilator-associated pneumonia

Definition

NICE defines ventilator-associated pneumonia (VAP) as 'pneumonia which develops 48 hours or more after intubation with an endotracheal or tracheostomy tube, and which was not present before':

- In the US up to 30% of ventilated ITU patients have a VAP.
- Patients who develop VAP have significantly longer duration of mechanical ventilation and ITU stay.
- Mortality is ↑ in patients by 30% if they have a VAP and can reach more than 70% if multiresistant pathogens are involved.

Diagnosis

VAP is a difficult diagnosis to make. Ideally clinical and radiological signs and positive microbiology will all coincide. Clinical signs may be non-specific, radiological signs may also be non-specific and lag behind clinical changes. Microbiological confirmation will be affected by:

- Sampling technique:
  - Sputum sample
  - Tracheal aspirate
  - Bronchoalveolar lavage
  - Protected specimen brush
- Recent antimicrobial therapy
- Pathogenicity of organisms
- Culture technique; quantitative vs non-quantitative.

A pragmatic approach used in Scottish ICUs is:

- The presence of new or persistent infiltrates on CXR and any 2 of:
  - Febrile >38°C
  - Leucocytosis or leukopenia (>11 or >3.5)
  - Purulent tracheobronchial secretions.

Aetiology

The micro-organisms responsible for VAP vary according to the population of patients in the ITU, the duration of hospital and ITU stays, and the diagnostic method used:

- Aerobic Gram-negative bacilli (GNB) are responsible for around 60% of VAP. The predominant GNB were *Pseudomonas aeruginosa* and *Acinetobacter* spp. followed by *Proteus, Escherichia coli, Klebsiella,* and *Haemophilus influenzae.*
- Gram-positive pneumonias are increasingly seen with *Staphylococcus aureus* being the most common.
- Polymicrobial infection in occurs in 20–50% of VAP.

Pre-disposing factors

- Prolonged antibiotic treatment increases the risk of superinfection with multiresistant organisms and delays the occurrence of nosocomial infection.
- ETT, reintubation, and tracheostomy: the presence of an ETT not only bypasses normal host defences but causes local trauma.

- NG tube, enteral feeding, and supine position.
- Respiratory equipment: ventilator circuits may be a source of bacteria responsible for VAP. The use of heat and moisture exchangers (HMEs) instead of heat humidifiers in suitable patients has been associated with a decrease in the risk of developing VAP

Prevention—VAP bundle

- *Elevation of the head of the bed to 35°.*
- *Daily 'sedation breaks'* reduce duration of mechanical ventilation.
- *Daily oral care* with chlorhexidine: dental plaque can be a reservoir for potential pathogens that cause VAP.
- *Peptic ulcer prophylaxis*: stress ulceration is the most common cause of GI bleeding in the critically ill and is associated with a 5-fold increase in mortality compared with those ITU patients without bleeding. Although there is a trend towards a lower pneumonia rate in patients treated with sucralfate rather than pH altering drugs, H_2 blockers were more effective in preventing peptic ulcer disease and so are the preferred agents.
- *DVT prophylaxis*: this is an appropriate intervention in all sedentary patients.

Further reading

Meade MO, Cook DJ, Guyatt GH, Slutsky AS, Arabi YM, Cooper DJ, et al.; Lung Open Ventilation Study Investigators. Ventilation strategy using low tidal volumes, recruitment maneuvers, and high positive end-expiratory pressure for acute lung injury and acute respiratory distress syndrome: a randomized controlled trial. *JAMA* 2008;299(6):637–45.

Mercat A, Richard J-CM Vielle B, Jaber S, Osman D, Diehl J-L, et al.; Expiratory Pressure (Express) Study Group. Positive end-expiratory pressure setting in adults with acute lung injury and acute respiratory distress syndrome: a randomized controlled trial. *JAMA* 2008;299(6):646–55.

Kidney

Acute kidney injury

Introduction

The principal functions of the kidney are:
- Regulation of body fluid volume and osmolality
- Excretion of metabolic end products and foreign substances
- Regulation of acid–base
- Production and secretion of enzymes and hormones (erythropoietin, renin, and 1,25 dihydroxyvitamin D_3).

In healthy subjects any change in body fluid volume, BP, or acid–base balance is corrected in a matter of hours, however in disease states these regulatory processes are disturbed.

The true incidence of acute kidney injury (AKI) in cardiac surgery is not clear, as there is significant variability in studies over how abrupt or severe the kidney dysfunction must be before it is defined as AKI. It is, however, a common complication of critical illness and an independent risk factor for postoperative death. The risk for death is proportional to the severity of kidney injury with mortality being as high as 50% in the general intensive care setting. Mortality is higher in patients with a sustained elevation of creatinine than in those who recover function.

All patients undergoing cardiac surgery are at risk of AKI either through their presenting illness or subsequent iatrogenic injury. Specific risk factors are listed in Table 13.1 and these should be considered prior to elective surgery. The most common pathogenesis of AKI following cardiac surgery is disrupted renal blood flow and the accepted prevention strategies are therefore:
- Appropriate IV volume expansion
- Optimization of CO
- Maintenance of renal blood flow and renal perfusion pressure.

'Renal dose dopamine'

There is no clinical benefit for its use in the prevention or treatment of AKI. Recent studies have shown it can worsen renal perfusion in patients with established AKI.

Furosemide infusion

Furosemide does not prevent the development of, or hasten the recovery from, AKI. Its inappropriate use can lead to intravascular hypovolaemia and worsening renal function. Loop diuretics can be used to correct volume overload in patients who are still responsive to treatment.

Key point: contrast-induced nephropathy

Identify patients at risk and carefully assess their fluid status. If indicated use pre- and postprocedure volume expansion with 0.9% sodium chloride or isotonic sodium bicarbonate. The use of N-acetyl cysteine is not recommended. Diuretics, NSAIDs, ACE inhibitors, and metformin should be withheld near the time of the procedure. As metformin is exclusively excreted by the kidneys, patients who develop AKI are at ↑ risk of lactic acidosis. If creatinine clearance is <60mL/min stop for 24 hours prior to contrast being given.

Table 13.1 Risk factors for the development of AKI following cardiac surgery

Preoperative	Intraoperative	Postoperative
Advanced age	Prolonged CPB time	Low CO syndrome
Female sex	Combined surgical procedures	Acute cardiac dysfunction
Chronic renal disease	Emergency surgery	Mediastinal haemorrhage
Diabetes mellitus	Previous cardiac surgery	Hypovolaemia
Chronic cardiac failure	Aortic clamp placement	Rhabdomyolysis
Aortic disease		Intra-abdominal hypertension
Peripheral vascular disease		Multiple organ dysfunction
Chronic liver disease		Drug nephrotoxicity
Genetic predisposition		
IABP		
Drug nephrotoxicity		

Key point: biomarkers in renal disease

Creatinine is currently the only biomarker of renal disease used in clinical practice. It is easily measured and specific for renal function; however, an acute decline in kidney function is not reflected by a rise in serum creatinine for several hours. For this reason urine output is used as a clinical monitor of renal function.

Further reading

Bellomo R, Chapman M, Finfer S, Hickling K, Myburgh J. Low-dose dopamine in patients with early renal dysfunction: a placebo-controlled randomised trial. ANZICS Clinical Trials Group. *Lancet* 2000;356:2139–43.

Friedrich JO, Adhikari N, Herridge MS, Beyene J. Meta-analysis: low dose dopamine increases urine output but does not prevent renal dysfunction or death. *Ann Intern Med* 2005;142:510–24.

Ho KM, Sheridan DJ. Meta-analysis of furosemide to prevent or treat AKI. *BMJ* 2006;333(7565):420–5.

Ho KM, Power BM. Benefits and risks of furosemide in AKI. *Anaesthesia* 2010;65:283–93.

Lauschke A, Teichgräber UK, Frei U, Eckardt KU. Low-dose dopamine worsens renal perfusion in patients with AKI. *Kidney Int* 2006;69:1669–74.

Definition and staging

The term acute renal failure implies that the function of the kidney is significantly deranged. Renal failure is a spectrum of disease from less severe forms of injury to more advanced injury where renal replacement therapy (RRT) may be required. A small increase in serum creatinine level is an independent predictor of morbidity and mortality and for this reason the term acute kidney injury (AKI) is now used to describe acute changes in renal function.

Table 13.2 KDIGO staging of AKI

Stage	Serum creatinine	Urine output
1	1.5–1.9 × baseline Or ≥0.3mg/dL (≥26.5µmol/L) increase	<0.5mL/kg/h for 6–12 hours
2	2.0–2.9 × baseline	<0.5mL/kg/h for ≥12 hours
3	3.0 × baseline Or Increase in serum creatinine to ≥4.0mg/dL (≥353.6µmol/L) Or Initiation of RRT Or In patients <18 years, decrease in eGFR to <35mL/min per 1.73m²	<0.3mL/kg/h for ≥24 hours Or Anuria for ≥12 hours

Kidney Disease: Improving Global Outcomes (KDIGO) Acute Kidney Injury Work Group. KDIGO 2012 Clinical Practice Guideline for Acute Kidney Injury. *Kidney Inter.*, Suppl. 2013: 3: 1–150, reproduced with permission.

AKI is generally defined as 'an abrupt and sustained decrease in kidney function'. The UK Renal Association recommends that the Acute Kidney Injury Network (AKIN) definition as adopted and refined by the Kidney Diseases: Improving Global Outcomes (KDIGO) International guideline group be used (Table 13.2).

AKI can be diagnosed when one of the following criteria is met:
- Serum creatinine rises by ≥26µmol/L from baseline within 48 hours *or*
- Serum creatinine rises ≥1.5× from baseline value which is known or presumed to have occurred within one week *or*
- Urine output documented <0.5mL/kg/hour for >6 consecutive hours.

General management

The aims of non-RRT management should be prevention of further kidney injury and supportive care to allow functional recovery. Management should begin with prompt diagnosis and correction of the underlying cause of renal injury. Although the most common pathologies in AKI post-cardiac surgery involve disruption of the renal blood flow all causes should be considered and excluded where appropriate. Sepsis is known to be a leading contributing factor to AKI in critical illness and should be diagnosed and treated promptly.

Clinical assessment general management measures
- Assess fluid balance and optimize haemodynamic status:
  - Clinical assessment—pulse, mean arterial blood pressure, capillary refill time, jugular or central venous pressure, Glasgow Coma Scale (GCS), acid–base balance, lactate, and serum albumin measurements
  - Ensure adequate fluid replacement
  - Consider the use of vasopressors or inotropes.

- Assess for complications of AKI:
  - Correct hypoxaemia if pulmonary oedema—continuous positive airway pressure (CPAP) or intubation and ventilation may be necessary until fluid can be removed with RRT
  - Recognize and treat hyperkalaemia
  - Assess for signs of uraemia—pericarditis, encephalopathy, drowsiness, seizures.
- Consider and correct reversible causes of AKI.
- Establish preoperative renal function.
- Exclude renal tract obstruction using ultrasonography.
- Identify and treat sepsis appropriately.
- *Stop and avoid nephrotoxic medication and dose adjust those drugs with renal clearance.*
- Treat metabolic acidosis.

Interpret a low urine output in the context of the patient's cardiovascular parameters:
- The oliguric patient may not be hypovolaemic.
- Urine output is influenced by the patient's cardiovascular parameters, hydration state, the use of diuretics, the presence of renal tract obstruction, and the stress response to injury.

Key point
Hyperkalaemia when associated with ECG change is a medical emergency.

Causes of AKI to consider
- Pre-renal (reduced renal perfusion):
  - Volume depletion, ↓ BP, ↓ CO, intrarenal vasoconstriction (drugs, radiographic contrast), hepatorenal syndrome.
- Renal or intrinsic:
  - Vascular (renal arterial disease, aortic atheroma/cholesterol emboli), nephrotoxins, infections, interstitial nephritis, accelerated phase hypertension, vasculitis, glomerulonephritis.
- Post-renal (obstruction):
  - Prostate hypertrophy, neurogenic bladder, intra ureteral obstruction (stones, tumour, thrombus, crystals), extra ureteral obstruction (tumour or retroperitoneal fibrosis).

Treatment of hyperkalaemia
Ensure stable cardiac rhythm:
- IV calcium gluconate or calcium carbonate if ECG changes—follow ALS guidelines.

Stop exogenous sources of potassium:
- Nutrition (oral/enteral/parenteral), potassium supplementation, IV fluid (e.g. Hartmann's solution).

Promote intracellular shift of potassium:
- IV Actrapid® 10 units in 50mL of 50% dextrose administered over 15–30 minutes:
  - Onset of action 15–30 minutes, max. effect 30–60 minutes, monitor blood glucose.
  - Repeat if continued hyperkalaemia.
- Nebulized salbutamol 5–10mg four times a day.
- Sodium bicarbonate:
  - Low pH leads to ↑ serum K^+ levels as K^+ shifts from the cellular to the vascular space.
  - The use of 500mL 1.26% $NaHCO_3$ may be indicated in the acidotic hyperkalaemic patient if fluid space allows but specialist advice should be sought.

Remove potassium from body:
- Restore urine output and recover renal function
- Oral (or rectal) calcium resonium 15g four times a day
- Consider RRT if refractory hyperkalaemia.

ECG changes in hyperkalaemia:
- Prolonged PR interval with flattening of loss of P waves
- Peaked T waves
- Widening of QRS interval
- Sine wave proceeding to ventricular fibrillation or asystole.

The ECG may be normal in life-threatening hyperkalaemia.

Fluid management
- The healthy adult requires 1.5–2.5L (25–35mL/kg/24 hours) water, around 70mmol/L sodium, and 40–80mmol/L of potassium per 24 hours.
- Fluid deficits occur without obvious fluid loss from vasodilation and altered capillary permeability.
- All fluid losses should be taken in to consideration including urine output, insensible losses, and fluid losses during theatre.
- The nature of fluid lost should be considered to enable appropriate choice of fluid replacement.
- 24-hour change in weight is the best measure of change in fluid balance.

It is recognized that excessive fluid administration with 0.9% sodium chloride can lead to sodium and chloride overload and hyperchloraemic metabolic acidosis. Balanced electrolyte solutions (Ringer's lactate or Hartmann's solution) should be used in preference to 0.9% sodium chloride in patients with AKI. Should, however, the patient be developing progressive AKI or hyperkalaemia treatment should change to non-potassium containing crystalloid solution.

Key point
The ability of critically ill patients to excrete excess Na and water is impaired placing them at ↑ risk of interstitial oedema.

Renal replacement therapy

RRT is an extracorporeal method of removing fluid and solutes from blood outside the body. During treatment blood comes in to contact with a semipermeable membrane where solute transfer occurs prior to it being returned to the patient. This can be carried out using intermittent (IRRT) or continuous (CRRT) techniques. In the acute setting IRRT is usually in the form of haemodialysis and CRRT is usually in the form of continuous veno-venous haemofiltration (CVVH) although hybrids of both techniques do exist.

IRRT—haemodialysis
- Solutes are removed by process of diffusion.
- Solute removal by this method is rapid and efficient.
- Fluid can be removed (ultrafiltration) by adjusting the pressures on the blood side of the semipermeable membrane.

CRRT—CVVH
- Solutes are removed by process of convection across a highly permeable filter.
- Convective solute removal is less efficient than diffusive but the continuous nature of the treatment compensates for this.
- The solute removal in CVVH is completely reliant on fluid removal therefore 'solute-free' fluid is replaced during the process either before (predilution) or after (postdilution) the blood comes in to contact with the semipermeable membrane

Consideration should be given to the type and dose of RRT chosen, the timing of initiation and discontinuation, access for RRT, and anticoagulation during RRT.

Type of RRT chosen
- CRRT offers no survival advantage over IRRT in patients with AKI.
- The type of RRT chosen does not influence the rate of renal recovery following AKI.
- CRRT is associated with a significantly ↑ risk of recurrent filter clotting compared to IRRT.
- Due to the continuous nature of CRRT there may be greater haemodynamic stability in patients with multiorgan failure and this is used in preference to IRRT in most ICUs.

Possible indications for urgent RRT
- Refractory hyperkalaemia >6.5mmol/L
- Refractory volume overload
- Refractory severe metabolic acidosis (pH <7.1)
- Signs of uraemia (e.g. pericarditis, neuropathy, seizures, or an otherwise unexplained decline in metal status)
- Certain drug and alcohol intoxications.

Indications for IRRT in preference to CRRT
- Drug poisoning: removal of specific toxins such as Li^+, theophyllines, etc.
- Bleeding risk: during CRRT blood is in contact with the extracorporeal circuit for longer and circuit clotting is more common, necessitating anticoagulation.
- Mobilization: rehabilitation and mobilization is difficult in patients receiving CRRT and in patients no longer confined to bed IRRT should be considered.

Initiation and discontinuation of RRT
There is lack of evidence to guide the optimal time to initiate RRT; however, for patients with multiorgan failure in the intensive care setting early initiation of RRT should be considered. When the urine output is ≥400mL/24 hours and the clinical condition of the patient is improving, discontinuation of RRT can be considered. Accurate assessment of fluid, electrolyte, and metabolic status is essential and RRT should be reconsidered if clinically indicated.

Dose of RRT
The dose of RRT can be altered by adjusting the blood flow, the area of the semipermeable membrane, or the duration of treatment. The prescribed dose should be assessed daily for continuous techniques and prior to each session for intermittent techniques.
- *IRRT*: the best evidence suggests patients should receive at least 3 sessions/week with delivered Kt/V value of 1.2. Most patients require daily or alternate day treatments to achieve this value.
- *CRRT*: the best evidence suggests patients should receive treatment doses equivalent to post dilution ultrafiltration rates ≥25mL/kg/hour.

Anticoagulation
Due to the requirement of extracorporeal blood flow in both IRRT and CRRT some form of anticoagulation is usually required to prevent thrombosis in the blood circuit. Type of RRT and risk of bleeding should be taken in to consideration when choosing type of anticoagulation.
- Heparin: bolus 1000–2000U at the start of RRT session followed by continuous infusion of 300–400U/hour. Aim for APPT in the venous limb 1.5–2 × control.
- Regional citrate anticoagulation: continuous infusion of isosmotic trisodium citrate solution (102mmol/L) in to the arterial side of the dialyser.
- Regional anticoagulation with protamine reversal: technically difficult with ↑ risk of rebound bleeding 2–4 hours post RRT.

Access
- In the acute setting access is veno-venous and the access site depends on the clinical condition of the patient.
- Ultrasound guidance should be used to aid placement of venous catheters and post-procedure CXR should confirm position.
- Internal jugular catheters should be 15–20cm in length and femoral catheters should be 20–25cm in length.

- Tunnelling of the venous catheter is desirable if RRT is likely to be prolonged (>3 weeks).

Complications of vascular access
- Catheter-related bacteraemia: the catheter should be reserved for extracorporeal treatment only to minimize the risk of catheter-related infection. The exit site should be carefully monitored and temporary access should be changed if there is clinical suspicion of catheter-related infection.
- Arrhythmia: insertion of internal jugular or subclavian catheters in the hyperkalaemic patient risks the guidewire touching the endocardium resulting in life-threatening and refractory arrhythmias.
- Clotting of dialysis catheter lumens: between periods of IRRT catheters should be locked with heparin (1000U/mL to the lumen volumes). This lock must be removed prior to recommencing RRT to avoid introducing heparin into the systemic circulation.

Complications of RRT
- Hypotension: can occur with both IRRT and CRRT. ↑ likelihood with high ultrafiltration rate, reduced LV function, and concurrent use of antihypertensive medications.
- Recirculation: caused when blood leaving the dialyser outlet returns to the inlet without having first passed through the peripheral bloodstream. This is more common with the use of femoral catheters and if the venous catheter used is an inadequate length.
- Infection: immune system dysregulation is multifactorial and patients with AKI have an ↑ susceptibility to infection.
- Cardiac arrhythmias: can occur with rapid change in serum electrolyte concentration. Carefully monitor and replace potassium, phosphate, and magnesium if necessary.
- Haemolysis.
- Air embolism.
- Rupture of the dialysis membrane: can lead to blood loss and entry of microorganisms to the bloodstream. Usually avoided by ensuring ultrafiltration rate (transmembrane pressure) is not too high.
- Reaction to dialysis membrane: rare complication. Clinical manifestations can vary from anaphylaxis to abdominal pain, fevers, or headaches.
- Disequilibrium syndrome: neurological signs and symptoms caused by cerebral oedema due to a rapid reduction in blood urea nitrogen. Onset of symptoms is usually during or shortly after IRRT, however the syndrome is now rare as RRT is initiated at an earlier stage.
- Transmission of blood-borne viruses.

Chronic kidney disease

Chronic kidney disease (CKD) is common in the general population and its prevalence is increasing. Cardiovascular disease is one of the most serious complications of CKD and cardiovascular disorders are the leading cause of death in patients with end-stage renal disease.

CKD is defined as:

- Kidney damage for ≥3 months, as defined by structural or functional abnormalities of the kidney, with or without ↓ GFR, manifest by *either*:
  - Pathological abnormalities *or*
  - Markers of kidney damage, including abnormalities in the composition of the blood or urine, or abnormalities in imaging tests
- GFR ≤60mL/min/1.73m^2 for ≥3 months with or without kidney damage (Table 13.3).

Influencing the progression of CKD

Slowing the progression of CKD reduces the morbidity and mortality associated. The *control of systemic hypertension* is the most effective intervention and current guidelines suggest:

- <140/90mmHg in patients with CKD
- <130/80mmHg in patients with CKD and diabetes or proteinuria (albumin:creatinine ratio (ACR) >70mg/mmol or protein:creatinine ratio (PCR) >100mg/mmol).

Other factors to consider are:

- Protein has a direct nephrotoxic effect. ACE inhibitors and angiotensin receptor blockers improve outcome in patients with proteinuric CKD.
- Poor diabetic control contributes to a faster rate of decline in diabetic nephropathy.
- Smoking is associated with more rapid progression of CKD.
- Superimposed AKI acts as a promoter for progression of underlying CKD.

Key point

AKI survivors with residual renal impairment should be managed according to local CKD guidelines. Discharge planning should encompass plans for CKD management and referral to specialist services if indicated. Refer to NICE CKD guideline for further information regarding appropriate follow-up.

Table 13.3 KDIGO staging of CKD

Stage	Description	GFR (mL/min/1.73m^2)
1	Kidney damage with normal or ↑ GFR	≥90
2	Kidney damage with mild ↓ GFR	60–89
3A	Moderate ↓ GFR	45–59
3B		30–44
4	Severe ↓ GFR	15–29
5	Kidney failure	<15 (or dialysis)

P suffix: the addition of p to a stage is used to denote the presence of proteinuria (this is defined as ACR ≥30mg/mmol or PCR ≥50mg/mmol).

T suffix: the addition of t to a stage indicates the patient has a renal transplant.

D suffix: the addition of d to a stage indicates the patient is on dialysis.

Kidney Disease: Improving Global Outcomes (KDIGO) CKD Work Group. KDIGO 2012 Clinical Practice Guideline for the Evaluation and Management of Chronic Kidney Disease. *Kidney Inter.*, Suppl. 2013; 3: 1–150, reproduced with permission.

Complications of CKD

- Cardiovascular disease: the traditional Framingham risk factors apply in CKD 1–3 but the Framingham tables significantly underestimate the risk of cardiovascular disease in patients with more advanced CKD. Statins reduce cardiovascular mortality in CKD stages 1–4. The role of statins in CKD5D patients is unclear and still under review.
- Hypertension: BP is a major risk factor for both cardiovascular and renal mortality. Dietary salt restriction should be suggested to all hypertensive patients with CKD. Target values are outlined as follows:
- Anaemia: consider the use of erythropoiesis stimulating agent (ESA) in anaemic patients with eGFR <25mL/min (<40mL/min in diabetic patients). Exclude causes other than renal impairment and ensure patients have adequate stores of iron, vitamin B$_{12}$ and folate prior to commencing ESA treatment. Aim for a target Hb of 11–12g/dL.
- Hyperparathyroidism and renal osteodystrophy: bone metabolism is disrupted in patients with moderate to severe CKD and accelerates vascular disease. In patients with CKD stage 3+ guidelines currently suggest serum calcium levels should be kept within normal limits, serum phosphate at or below 1.8mmol/L and PTH below 2–3 × the upper limit of normal. Specialist advice should be sought in patients who have evidence of renal bone disease.
- Metabolic acidosis: CKD stage 3+.
- Infection: alterations in both cellular and humoral immunity occur leading to a significant ↑ susceptibility of infection. This worsens with progression of uraemia and stage of CKD.
- Malnutrition: anorexia and nausea are commonly found in patients with advancing CKD. Vitamin supplementation may be required.

Chapter 14

127

Gastrointestinal

Gastrointestinal complications after cardiac surgery

Gastrointestinal (GI) complications after cardiac operations are infrequent (0.3–3%) but serious. The overall mortality from GI complications ranges from 11–72% and has not ↓ significantly during the last two decades. GI conditions range from mild, but troublesome, complications like ileus to devastating complications such as bowel ischaemia and liver failure.

Common complications

- GI bleeding (33%), mortality 20%
- Mesenteric ischaemia (14%), mortality 50–100%
- Pancreatitis (11%), mortality 20%
- Acute cholecystitis (9%), mortality 26%
- Perforated peptic ulcer (5%), mortality 36%
- Liver failure (2%), mortality 56%.

Risk factors

Numerous risk factors for GI complications have been reported and can be classified as pre-, intra-, and postoperative. The factors that have been identified on multivariate analysis are:

- Preoperative: age >70 years, low CO (22-fold ↑ risk), peripheral vascular disease, reoperative surgery and chronic renal failure
- Intra- and postoperative: ↑ need for blood transfusions, prolonged CPB, dysrhythmias (17-fold ↑ risk), IABP.

These factors are general markers of how unwell these patients are as well as proxy markers for the complexity of their surgery. Mesenteric ischaemia is often the final part of a tragic tale of organ dysfunction in patients who likely would have died from circulatory failure anyway, with or without GI complications.

The cause of GI complications is still unknown but most theories implicate low CO resulting in visceral hypoperfusion and ischaemia. This process triggers a hormonal stress response and leads to a mediator-driven systemic inflammatory response.

The role of CPB in the aetiology of GI complications is controversial. One randomized trial showed a significant decrease of GI complications in coronary bypass off-pump vs on-pump. These results have not been duplicated and most studies found no difference with regard to GI complications, gastric mucosal oxygenation, or superior mesenteric arterial blood flow when comparing on-pump with off-pump CABG.

Other perioperative interventions have been shown to reduce the incidence of GI complications like stress-ulcer prophylaxis and goal-directed haemodynamic therapy and even intraoperative manoeuvres like epi-aortic scanning prior to clamping shows promise.

Ischaemic bowel

Occurs after 0.16% of all cardiac operations and has a mortality of 50% on average but may be as high as 100% in some reports. The patients are commonly on mechanical ventilation and sedated, thus making the usual signs of abdominal pain and tenderness unreliable. Furthermore, many patients with multiple organ dysfunction in intensive care develop distended and tender abdomens with ileus making it a diagnostic challenge to identify the patient with ischaemic bowel.

The onset is usually gradual and non-specific with Ileus, abdominal distension, ↑ NG output, ↑ need for organ support, raised inflammatory markers, hyperkalaemia, unexplained lactic acidosis, and lower GI bleeding. All of these are non-specific and contribute to a delay in diagnosis with ↑morbidity and mortality.

Mesenteric ischaemia can be occlusive, non-occlusive and rarely due to mesenteric venous thrombosis.

- Non-occlusive mesenteric ischaemia (NOMI) is more common and thought to be secondary to hypoperfusion and the use of vasopressor drugs. The onset is slower and more gradual than occlusive ischaemia. If suspected and the patient does not need urgent laparotomy for bowel necrosis (as indicated by severe acidosis, peritonitis, CT findings) the diagnosis can be made with mesenteric angiography showing the characteristic 'string of sausages' signs due to constrictions in the mesenteric arteries.
- Management in the early stages include: broad-spectrum antibiotics, aggressive resuscitation to maximize mesenteric blood flow, NG tube decompression, and intra-arterial papaverine infusion (bolus of 60mg followed by continuous infusion of 0.7mg/kg per hour) through the intra-arterial catheter placed into the SMA during arteriography.
- If bowel necrosis is already established urgent laparotomy is required.
- Occlusive mesenteric ischaemia may be caused by emboli or thrombus formation and has sudden onset with acute clinical deterioration. Diagnosis is commonly made on CT angiography. Management is usually operative with laparotomy, revascularization, and resection of necrosed bowel. Alternatives to mesenteric bypass like embolectomy, angioplasty, stenting, and thrombolytics have been reported but their use in post-cardiac surgery (especially thrombolytics) needs to be established.
- Mesenteric venous thrombosis leads to swelling of the bowel and eventual arterial occlusion. The diagnosis is made on contrast-enhanced CT scan and management includes urgent anticoagulation.

The outcome of mesenteric ischaemia is dependent on early diagnosis which requires a high index of suspicion and a willingness to aggressively investigate and explore patients early. The principles of operative surgery are as follows:

- Revascularize before resection to minimize bowel loss
- Liberal use of second-look laparotomy.

Where there is agreement that bowel ischaemia is part of progressive and irreversible organ dysfunction syndrome due to poor perfusion, a multidisciplinary decision (along with relatives) should be made to limit intervention in a patient who is deemed to be in an end of life situation.

Acute pancreatitis

Any patient with abdominal symptoms and signs post-cardiac surgery should have a s-amylase test. Hyperamylasemia occurs in 30–40% of patients after cardiac surgery, but only 1–3% of these have clinical pancreatitis. Amylase may also be raised in numerous other conditions including perforated viscus and ischaemic bowel. Contrast-enhanced CT should always be performed to confirm the diagnosis and rule out other conditions that may require urgent operative intervention.

Hyperamylasemia on its own does not warrant any specific treatment whereas the presence of clinical and radiological evidence of pancreatitis needs supportive management:

- Adjust IV fluid therapy to meet the ↑ demands of massive retroperitoneal fluid sequestration.
- No longer should 'bowel rest' be employed. Enteral feeding (normal oral route, NG, or nasojejunal is acceptable) should always be encouraged above total parenteral nutrition (TPN). The route should be adjusted to compensate for vomiting, gastric stasis, and ileus which commonly occur.
- Routine antibiotics are not recommended in the absence of necrosis.
- Repeat CT if condition deteriorates to diagnose and manage pancreatic necrosis and infected necrosis, increasingly by radiological and percutaneous drainage rather than open necrosectomy.

Acute cholecystitis

Cholecystitis typically occurs 5–15 days postoperatively and rarely presents with classical symptoms of right upper quadrant pain. Instead, patients develop SIRS and/or ↑ unexplained haemodynamic instability. Diabetics are at ↑ risk and do not present typical clinical signs. As opposed to cholecystitis in the general population, at least half of cases post cardiac surgery have acalculous disease and approximately half of patients will have gangrenous cholecystitis. It is therefore important to intervene before gangrene and perforation occurs (within 24 hours of onset of symptoms) as the mortality rises sharply thereafter.

Management has to be individualized:

- Percutaneous cholecystostomy (at the bedside under ultrasound guidance) is an option for unstable patients in the absence of perforation.
- Cholecystectomy, partial or total is the treatment of choice and can be done open or laparoscopically. Large drains are recommended as cystic duct/gallbladder remnant bile leaks are not uncommon. This can be managed with endoscopic retrograde cholangiopancreatography (ERCP) and temporary biliary stenting.

Liver failure and hyperbilirubinaemia

After cardiac surgery up to 25% of patients may experience a rise in bilirubin, usually peaking on the 1st or 2nd postoperative day with a mortality rate of around 4%. Liver failure, as defined by the loss of synthetic and metabolic function of the liver (↓ production of clotting factors and albumin) and the development of hepatic encephalopathy, occurs in <0.1% of cardiac patients but carries a mortality rate of >50%. It is often a manifestation of multiple organ dysfunction syndrome, but may be drug induced.

Management includes:
- Improving haemodynamics and liver perfusion
- Stopping hepatotoxic drugs
- Liver screen for underlying hepatic and haematological disease
- Ultrasound and CT to rule out biliary obstruction, portal venous obstruction, and hepatic vein thrombosis.

GI complications after cardiac surgery are fortunately rare as they carry a significant mortality rate. It remains one of the greatest clinical and diagnostic challenges in cardiac ITU. A general surgeon should be involved early as a delay in diagnosis and treatment has a high mortality. A team approach to management is ideal to ensure that patients receive timely intervention when needed but also, and just as important, that patients for whom death is inevitable do not suffer pointless and frankly cruel interventions in the final stages of their lives.

Investigating the acute abdomen

Post-cardiac surgery patients in ICU can present with abdominal symptoms in a variety of ways. The presentation may be obvious with acute onset of symptoms and signs in a patient who is not sedated and on minimal supportive therapy. It is easier to diagnose these patients more accurately with clinical examination, laboratory, and imaging investigations. On the other end of the spectrum, patients may be profoundly unwell with multiple organ dysfunction on an array of life support therapies with subtle and insidious signs of GI disturbance. These patients remain one of the greatest diagnostic challenges and often the correct diagnosis is only made at laparotomy or postmortem.

Clinical history and examination

Post-cardiac surgery patients are often sedated and ventilated. Symptoms are therefore not reported and physical signs can be unreliable and may only become obvious at a late and irreversible stage. That said, there is no reliable laboratory or imaging indicator (especially for mesenteric ischaemia). The only objective 'test' is laparotomy. Therefore, clinical examination by an experienced acute GI surgeon is still the only, although imperfect, modality to essentially decide on the need for surgery.

A careful history should include:
- Nature of cardiac surgery, intra- and postoperative course, time elapsed since operation
- Previous history of GI disease, abdominal surgery
- 'Subtle' signs of GI complications such as abdominal distension, non-absorption of feed, and ↑ NG output
- Deterioration of organ dysfunction for no other apparent reason.

Physical examination
- Focal tenderness is a more indicative sign than generalized tenderness.
- Unless peritonitis is present, abdominal examination may remain unremarkable.
- In the presence of equivocal findings, repeated examination by the same surgeon is invaluable as it is often subtle changes that are not communicated that are the most helpful.

Laboratory test

No laboratory test can reliably establish or eliminate the diagnosis of mesenteric ischaemia. The following blood tests are used as an adjunct:
- Arterial blood gas—pH
- s-lactate
- s-phosphate
- s-amylase
- Liver function tests (LFTs)
- Full blood count (FBC)—white cell count.

As expected, most of these will be abnormal in patients who are often haemodynamically unstable and have a high incidence of organ dysfunction. Acid–base status, s-lactate, and s-phosphate are altered by renal replacement therapy.

Imaging

- Abdominal X-ray: findings are usually non-specific, e.g. dilated loops of bowel, thickened bowel wall, and ascites which are late findings. It can be normal in up to 25%. Its role is more to rule out perforation and bowel obstruction.
- Ultrasound and mesenteric duplex Doppler is not very useful in the acute setting as distended gas-filled loops of bowel degrade and obscure the images.
- Mesenteric angiogram is still regarded as the gold standard but its use in critically ill patients is limited because of its invasive, time-consuming nature and the need for high doses of contrast. In selected, stable patients without established infarction it may be useful and even therapeutic allowing interventions such as stents, angioplasty, and in the case of NOMI, intra-arterial infusion of papaverine.
- CT: multidetector row CT has overcome most of the limitations of earlier scanners with faster scanner and thinner collimation. Sophisticated post processing can render images of the mesenteric vasculature comparable to angiography. In the critically ill patient, often with poor CO and renal impairment, the constraints in accurate timing and dose of contrast reduces the sensitivity and specificity (correlates with laparotomy findings in <50% of cases where mesenteric ischaemia is suspected). It is, however, useful to diagnose pancreatitis, bowel obstruction, cholecystitis, and perforation.

Early aggressive investigation of patients who show clinical and radio-logical signs of paralytic ileus with one or more of the following signs should be promptly investigated with high-quality CT and/or mesenteric arteriography:

- No bowel movement 3 days after cardiac surgery despite laxatives
- Bloated, distended abdomen
- High output from NG tube
- Non-absorption of feed.

Ultimately, the only objectively reliable 'investigation' is laparotomy and this should be offered early in patients with suspicious findings. In the absence of frank dead bowel it may be difficult, even at laparotomy, to distinguish mesenteric ischaemia. Limited reports of diagnostic laparoscopy found it safe and accurate in this setting.

Gastrointestinal bleeding

GI bleeding occurs in 0.3–1% of post-cardiac surgery patients and accounts for about 33% of GI complications.

Upper GI bleeding

The mortality rate of bleeding from the upper GI tract after cardiac surgery is high (15–35%) and not dissimilar to the mortality seen in other hospitalized patients who bleed. Acute stress ulceration due to ischaemia/reperfusion injury is the most common cause, further complicated by the ubiquitous use of anticoagulants and/or antiplatelet drugs. Another risk factor is prolonged ventilation. There is some evidence that a prior history of GI bleeding/ulceration increases risk. Helicobacter pylori does not appear to be associated with stress ulceration in post-cardiac surgery patients.

The bleeding lesion is acid related in 75% of cases: gastritis, gastric ulcer, duodenal ulcer, and erosive oesophagitis. Less common lesions include varices (rare in cardiac surgery patients), Mallory–Weiss syndrome and vascular lesions, e.g. Dieulafoy lesions.

The majority of upper GI bleeding is self-limiting. Significant, ongoing bleeding needs urgent management.

Principles of management
- Resuscitation. Adequate haemodynamic stability and transfusion of blood products is obviously important.
- Prophylactic antibiotics. Therapeutic endoscopic procedures cause transient bacteraemia putting patients with prosthetic valves etc. at risk for endocarditis.
- Anticoagulant, antiplatelet therapy should be stopped and coagulopathy should be corrected.
- Endoscopy. The timing depends on the situation. Stable patients need an urgent endoscopy to establish and treat the source of bleeding. Unstable patients despite adequate resuscitation need intubating (if not already intubated) and endoscopy should take place as part of the resuscitation.
- Endoscopic haemostasis is the treatment of choice and >90% successful in stopping the bleeding. It may be necessary to lavage the stomach to remove blood clots to identify the source of bleeding. The prokinetic effect of IV erythromycin is a proven way of reducing blood clots in the stomach. Combination therapy (adrenaline injection with either heater probe or haemoclips) is superior to monotherapy. When faced with an adherent clot to the ulcer base this should be removed to treat the underlying lesion.
- IV PPI infusion post endostasis reduces the risk of rebleeding. Omeprazole 80mg IV followed by an infusion of 8mg/hour for 72 hours. This is followed by 20mg of oral omeprazole for at least 8 weeks or indefinite maintenance for patients on non-steroidal anti-inflammatories.
- Enteral nutrition should be resumed as soon as bleeding has stopped and the patient is stable and able to tolerate feeding.

- Where endostasis fails, laparotomy and suturing of the bleeding point is the only option. This is a self-selecting group with a higher mortality approaching 45%.

Lower GI bleeding

Lower GI bleeding in the CICU setting is associated with a 17–20% mortality. The most common causes remain diverticular bleeding and angiodysplastic lesions. Bleeding from these lesions is self-limiting in >90% of cases, provided anticoagulant and antiplatelet therapy is stopped. Other causes are colitis (mostly ischaemic), neoplasia, and anorectal bleeding. It must be kept in mind that up to 10% of lower GI bleeding is actually bleeding from an upper GI source.

Management

- Resuscitation and transfusion.
- Correct coagulopathy.
- Rule out upper GI source especially if massive bleed causing haemodynamic instability.
- All patients should have colonoscopy after proper bowel prep in the weeks to come once discharged from ICU and able to tolerate the procedure. The main purpose is to rule out underlying colorectal malignancy.
- In the minority who do not stop bleeding the options are:
  - Colonoscopy in unprepared bowel which is difficult yielding a diagnosis in 70–80%.
  - It may be possible to use endostasis techniques.
  - Angiography or CT angiography to establish the bleeding point followed by segmental resection.
  - In desperate cases a subtotal colectomy may be the only viable option.

Nutrition in CICU

Introduction

It is estimated that 10–40% of all patients in hospital are undernourished. In addition, critically ill patients lose approximately 5–10% of skeletal muscle mass per week during their ICU stay. It is therefore recommended that critical care patients are fed to counteract catabolic state.

There is a lot of literature on nutrition in critically ill patients, but few high-quality trials. These recommendations are based on guidelines produced by the Canadian Critical Care Network, by ESPEN (the European Society for Parenteral and Enteral Nutrition) and NICE.

Requirements

- 20–30kcal/kg body weight increasing to 25–30kcal/kg
- Nitrogen 0.17–0.2g/kg body weight (1–1.25g protein/kg).

This does not allow for age, sex, obesity and metabolic state and so an individual patient's requirements should be assessed by a dietitian.

Feeding

The provision of nutrition should be started within 24–48 hours of admission to CICU if the patient is not expected to become established on oral diet within 3 days (ESPEN). Enteral tube feeding uses the physiological route, is cheap, and is generally safe. In the presence of a functioning GI tract it is the preferred route of nutrition support.

Enteral nutrition

The simplest technique is via NG tube:
- Reducing the risk of aspiration:
  - NG tube position should be confirmed on placement and checked regularly
  - 45° head-up position
- Promoting enteral feed:
  - Check gastric emptying aspirate from NG tube 4- to 6-hourly. Acceptable volume of aspirates vary as per local policy (up to 400mL), if able return some/all aspirate to maintain gut function.

High aspirate is a common reason why patients do not receive full prescribed volume of feed therefore consider the following:
- Reduced use of opiates.
- The use of prokinetic agents—metoclopramide 10mg four times a day and/or erythromycin. There is not a standard regimen for erythromycin when used as a prokinetic agent. With IV erythromycin, satisfactory outcomes have been achieved with doses of 300mg daily in divided doses, with 250mg four times a day, and with single doses of 70mg and 200mg.
- Ensure that feed rate is not reduced based on one aspirate, monitor trend and review rate in line with clinical assessment—abdomen, regurgitation, nausea, and vomiting.

If aspirates prevent adequate feeding consider post-pyloric feeding with a naso-jejunostomy tube. To ensure correct positioning this may require endoscopic or radiological placement.

Administration

Start feed at low rate (25–30mL/hour); if tolerated increase in 25–30mL increments until target rate met.

Fluid requirements should be decided by medical staff. Depending on volume available for feeding, standard (1.0kcal/mL) or high-energy and/or protein feeds (1.2–2.0kcal/mL) can be used.

Parenteral nutrition

If enteral feeding is not achieving nutrition targets, consider early conversion to parenteral feeding. Where available the multidisciplinary nutrition team will assess and advise.

Consider:

- When the GI tract is not functional or cannot be accessed
- When the patient's nutrient needs are greater than those which can be met through the GI tract.

Parenteral nutrition (PN) may be delivered through peripheral venous access in the short term. Ideally it is delivered into a central vein through a peripherally inserted central catheter (PICC), a dedicated central venous feeding line, or through a dedicated lumen of a central line. Pharmacy will advise on PN bags available. Asepsis must be strictly adhered to.

Administration

Options are 'All-in-one' mixtures with added electrolytes and micro-nutrients or individually tailored PN bags:

- Some of the energy should come from lipid sources but there is paucity of evidence to suggest any particular lipid formulations. Caution should be applied when other lipid containing infusions are also in use (e.g. propofol). Lipid infusion is safe at rates up to 1.5g/kg/day.
- Glucose can be given at 4–5g/kg/day. In all critically ill patients avoid hyperglycaemia (blood glucose >10mmol/L) by minimizing IV dextrose and using insulin administration when necessary.
- Nitrogen requirements should be met in standard solutions.
- Estimate electrolyte requirements based on clinical condition and discuss with pharmacy regarding additions to PN bag.
- Micronutrient solutions providing vitamins and trace elements should be added by pharmacy prior to dispensing.

Assess volume requirements and infusion rate. PN should be infused using a volumetric pump normally over 24 hours.

Monitoring

Nutritional support needs to be monitored to assess efficacy and detect any complications. The measurements and their frequency depend on the severity of the patient's illness and the stage of feeding.

- Biochemistry—urea & electrolytes (U&Es) daily; glucose at least once daily; bone profile daily, once stable twice weekly; LFTs twice weekly.
- Fluid balance—fluid balance daily, patient weight daily.

- Nutritional status—weight and nitrogen balance weekly. Interpret both with care re: fluid balance. There is wide individual response.
- Trace elements and vitamin status—inflammatory status of patient (C-reactive protein (CRP)) should be assessed before requesting nutrition screen as results are difficult to interpret. Discuss with biochemistry department.

Further reading

Kreymann KG, Berger MM, Deutz NE, Hiesmayr M, Jolliet P, Kazandjiev G, et al. ESPEN guidelines on enteral nutrition: intensive care. Clin Nutr 2006;25:210–23.

National Institute for Health and Clinical Excellence (NICE). Nutritional Support for Adults Oral Nutritional Support, Enteral Tube Feeding and Parenteral Nutrition. Clinical Guideline 32. London: NICE; 2006.

Todorovic V, Mickelwright A (eds) on behalf of the Parenteral and Nutrition Group of the British Dietetic Association. A Pocket Guide to Clinical Nutrition, 4th ed. London: Parenteral and Enteral Nutrition Group; 2011.

Nervous system

Delirium

- Delirium is an acute and fluctuating change in cognition characterized by inattention with either a fluctuating level of consciousness or disorganized thinking.
- Part of the spectrum of neuropsychiatric changes commonly seen after cardiac surgery and often referred to as 'pump-head' or post-perfusion syndrome.
- Significant crossover with stroke in terms of risk factors, pathophysiology, and clinical presentation.

Incidence

- Incidence varies depending on the technique used for measurement, the age group assessed and the type of surgery (Table 15.1).

Table 15.1 Incidence of delirium varies depending on the measurement technique, age group, and type of surgery

Measurement technique	Patient age group	Surgery	Incidence
Daily clinical assessment	Adult patients	CABG on CPB	7.9%
		CABG off CPB	2.3%
		Valve or combined	11.2%
Interviews with nurse	<65 years	CABG	3%
	>65 years	CABG	9%
Validated diagnostic tool	>60 years	CABG, valve, combined	52%

Risk factors

- Multiple factors have been associated with ↑ risk of delirium post cardiac surgery (Table 15.2).

Pathophysiology

Aetiology of delirium is complex and involves the interaction of the risk factors in Table 15.2 with:

- Pharmacological effects (including anaesthesia, analgesia and drug withdrawal)
- Ischaemia (secondary to embolization and hypoperfusion)
- Inflammation and infection
- Environmental factors (overstimulation and sleep deprivation)
- Pathophysiological effects of CPB are implicated in the aetiology of delirium. However, delirium remains a problem following off-pump surgery
- Underlying neuropathological mechanisms are poorly understood but there is evidence that an imbalance of central neurotransmission including a reduction in cholinergic and an increase in dopaminergic neurotransmission is likely to be important.

Table 15.2 Risk factors for delirium post cardiac surgery

Preoperative	Intra and postoperative
↑ age	Urgent operation
Severe cardiac disease (EF <30%, cardiogenic shock)	Type of operation (valvular or combined surgery)
Systemic vascular disease (hypertension, cerebro-vascular disease,[a] peripheral vascular disease)	Prolonged operation and CPB
Other medical conditions (respiratory disease, AF, renal disease, diabetes)	Hypoperfusion
Impaired cognition[a] or existing depression[a]	Large volume transfusion
Low albumin[a]	Prolonged mechanical ventilation
Alcohol excess	Hypoxia
Smoking	

[a]Risk factors included in a validated preoperative prediction model for postoperative delirium.

Clinical features

- Delirium can be hyperactive (restless, agitated, aggressive), hypoactive (withdrawn, quiet, sleepy) or mixed (Table 15.3).
- Hypoactive or mixed delirium accounts for 75% of cases and has been associated with worse prognosis due to diagnostic delay.
- If delirium is suspected in a patient in critical care, assessment should be done using the validated tool CAM-ICU (Fig. 15.1).
- Without the use of an appropriate assessment tool, up to 75% of cases of ICU delirium are missed.

Table 15.3 Richmond Agitation Sedation Scale (RASS)

RASS	Term	Description
+4	Combative	Overtly combative or violent; immediate danger to staff
+3	Very agitated	Pulls on or removes tube(s) or catheter(s) or has aggressive behaviour toward staff
+2	Agitated	Frequent non-purposeful movement or patient-ventilator dyssynchrony
+1	Restless	Anxious or apprehensive but movements not aggressive or vigorous
0	Alert and calm	
−1	Drowsy	Not fully alert, but has sustained (more than 10 seconds) awakening, with eye contact, to voice
−2	Light sedation	Briefly (less than 10 seconds) awakens with eye contact to voice
−3	Moderate sedation	Any movement (but no eye contact) to voice
−4	Deep sedation	No response to voice, but any movement to physical stimulation
−5	Unarousable	No response to voice or physical stimulation

Reprinted with permission of the American Thoracic Society. Copyright © 2014 American Thoracic Society. The Richmond Agitation–Sedation Scale: Validity and Reliability in Adult Intensive Care Unit Patients' Curtis N. Sessler, Mark S. Gosnell, Mary Jo Grap, Gretchen M. Brophy, Pam V. O'Neal, Kimberly A. Keane, Eljim P. Tesoro and R. K. Elswick, Am. J. Respir. Crit. Care Med. Official Journal of the American Thoracic Society. 2002; 166: 1338–1344. http://ajrccm.atsjournals.org/content/166/10/1338.full.

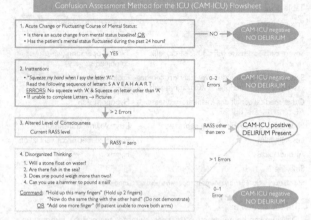

Figure 15.1 Confusion assessment method for the ICU. Copyright © 2002, E. Wesley Ely, MD, MPH and Vanderbilt University, all rights reserved.

Investigation

- Perform thorough physical examination and review medications.
- Further investigation will be guided by clinical exam but should include bloods (FBC, U&E, LFT, glucose, Ca), ECG, and sepsis screen as a minimum.
- Cerebral imaging is unlikely to affect clinical management in the delirious patient in the absence of focal neurological signs. In addition, sedation may be required to facilitate imaging and can prolong the course of delirium.

Prevention

- A number of strategies to prevent neurological complications in cardiac surgery have been proposed (see 🕮 Neurological complications of cardiac surgery, p. 144).
- There is a randomized trial that found a reduced incidence of delirium comparing the α-2 agonist dexmedetomidine with benzodiazepines for ICU sedation.
- The 'ABCDE' bundle has been proposed as an evidence-based structured approach to minimizing brain dysfunction in mechanically ventilated ICU patients.
  - *A*wakening and *B*reathing *C*oordination involving spontaneous awakening trials combined with spontaneous breathing trials
  - *D*elirium monitoring using a validated assessment tool
  - *E*xercise and *E*arly mobility.

- NICE guideline on delirium advocates a multi-component intervention package in patients identified as at risk of delirium. Care should be taken to:
  - Provide an appropriately stimulating environment and reorientate as required
  - Avoid hypoxia
  - Ensure adequate hydration and avoid constipation
  - Identify and treat infection
  - Ensure adequate nutrition
  - Identify and treat pain
  - Avoid sleep disturbance
  - Avoid sensory deprivation by ensuring visual and hearing aids are working
  - Encourage early mobilization
  - Review medications and consider side effects.

Treatment

- Primary strategy is to identify and treat any underlying causes.
- If the patient is distressed then use verbal and non-verbal de-escalation techniques.
- If these are ineffective then consider a short course of haloperidol or second-generation olanzapine, quetiapine, risperidone starting at the lowest appropriate dose.
- Alpha-2 agonists are commonly used as second-line treatment. Dexmedetomidine is not licensed in the UK so clonidine is the drug of choice.

Outcomes

- Following cardiac surgery, cerebral complications including delirium have been associated with ↑ ICU and hospital stay and ↑in-hospital mortality.
- There is evidence that delirium post coronary artery bypass surgery increases the risk of late mortality up to 10 years.
- However, a recent study has shown no ↑ rates of postoperative cognitive decline at 3 months post CABG compared to total hip joint replacement or coronary angiography done without general anaesthesia.

Further reading

Curtis N, Sessler MS, Gosnell MJ, Grap GM, Brophy PV, O'Neal KA, *et al*. The Richmond Agitation–Sedation Scale: validity and reliability in adult intensive care unit patients. *Am J Respir Crit Care Med* 2002;166:1338–44.

Ely EW, Inouye SK, Bernard GR, Gordon S, Francis J, May L, *et al*. Delirium in mechanically ventilated patients: validity and reliability of the confusion assessment method for the intensive care unit (CAM-ICU). *JAMA* 2001;286:2703–10.

Rudolph JL, Jones RN, Levkoff SE, Rockett C, Inouye SK, Sellke FW, *et al*. Derivation and validation of a preoperative prediction rule for delirium after cardiac surgery. *Circulation* 2009;119:229–36.

Young J, Murthy L, Westby M, Akunne A, O'Mahony R; Guideline Development Group. Diagnosis, prevention, and management of delirium: summary of NICE guidance. *BMJ* 2010;341:c3704.

Neurological complications of cardiac surgery

Introduction

Neurological complications are a major source of morbidity and mortality following cardiac surgery. Present as a spectrum of overlapping disorders, which can be classified as: stroke, encephalopathy (often presenting as neurocognitive deficits including delirium), and peripheral neuropathy.

Stroke

- Stroke is the rapid onset of neurological deficit secondary to infarction or haemorrhage and lasting >24 hours.
- Majority of strokes following cardiac surgery are secondary to infarction.

Incidence

- Significant variation in the reported incidence of perioperative stroke in cardiac surgery.
- Table 15.4 presents data from a large cohort from a single institution and from the Society of Thoracic Surgeons National Adult Cardiac Surgery Database (STS NCD).
- Surgery involving combined procedures, the mitral valve, or the aorta has a particularly high risk of perioperative stroke.

Table 15.4 High variation in the incidence of stroke demonstrated in data derived from a single institution and from the STS NCD

Cardiac surgical procedure	STS NCD	Single institution
CABG	1.4%	4.1%
Valve	1.6%	3.1%
CABG/Valve	2.9%	7.9%

Risk factors

- With the exception of female sex, largely represent risk factors for systemic vascular disease: ↑ age, hypertension, diabetes, chronic kidney disease, peripheral vascular disease, previous history of cerebrovascular disease, known atherosclerosis of the ascending aorta or carotids, AF.
- Patients presenting with a recent MI, unstable angina, or moderate to severe LV systolic dysfunction are at ↑ risk.
- Several prediction models exist that account for the additive effect of risk factors in an individual patient.

Pathophysiology

- Stroke can be classified as intraoperative or postoperative depending on whether the deficit is present immediately on waking from anaesthesia.
- Aetiology is likely multifactorial but a primary mechanism is thought to be atheromatous embolism arising from the ascending aorta.
- Cerebral emboli of particulate matter also arise from cardiac thrombi, severely calcified valves, and carotid artery atherosclerosis.
- Gaseous emboli arise from open cardiac chambers, vascular cannulation sites, or arterial anastomoses.
- Cerebral hypoperfusion may contribute to intraoperative stroke by reducing the washout out of embolic material from watershed areas of brain at the borders of vascular territories.
- The inflammatory process and hypercoagulability may contribute to postoperative stroke.

Clinical features

- Depend on the location of brain injury and whether the ischemia is regional or global.
- Any combination of hemiparesis, ataxia, hemisensory loss, visual disturbance, dysarthria, dysphasia, or effects on consciousness or cognition.

Investigation

- Neuroimaging will confirm the diagnosis of ischaemic or haemorrhagic stroke. Perform routine investigations to identify aetiological factors and exclude alternative causes of neurological impairment.
- ECG—AF, other arrhythmia.
- Echocardiogram—intracardiac thrombus, new valve pathology.
- Bloods—include FBC, coagulation screen, U&Es, calcium, glucose, LFTs, and thyroid function tests as first line.
- Imaging should be performed as soon as possible to exclude haemorrhage.
- CT will identify about 50% of infarcts.
- Magnetic resonance imaging (MRI) is the technique of choice. Diffusion-weighted imaging can detect acute ischemic events related to microemboli. It is more likely to demonstrate multiple lesions in a watershed pattern of distribution than T2 or FLAIR imaging.

Prevention

- A number of strategies to prevent neurological complications including stroke have been proposed. Evidence supporting individual neuroprotective techniques is sparse.
- Preoperative—combine thorough preoperative assessment with the use of scoring systems to identify high-risk patients and thus focus resources.
- Off-pump surgery—no consensus regarding the avoidance of CPB to reduce the incidence of neurological complications but off-pump surgery can be considered.

- Surgical technique—epiaortic ultrasound guidance and 'no touch technique' may help to reduce aortic atheroma embolization. Use of aortic cannulae with improved flow characteristics and with filters may be beneficial.
- CPB—membrane oxygenators reduce emboli compared to bubble oxygenators. No evidence to support pH over α-stat management or pulsatile over non-pulsatile flow. Targeting of higher haematocrit (>27%) and higher MAP (minimum >50mmHg) may be beneficial. Hypothermia used for neuroprotection despite conflicting evidence.
- Multimodal neuromonitoring—optimization of intraoperative care using a combination of cerebral monitors such as transcranial Doppler, electroencephalogram, and cerebral oximetry using near-infrared spectroscopy has been suggested. Cerebral desaturation has been shown to correlate with neurological impairment but protocolized treatment of desaturations did not improve outcome.
- Pharmacotherapy—no evidence to support the use of any agent for pharmacological neuroprotection. Thiopentone is often used during deep hypothermic circulatory arrest.
- Combined carotid endarterectomy and cardiac surgery—there is no evidence that this approach reduces the risk of stroke in patents with carotid stenosis and outcomes may be worse.

Treatment

- Antiplatelet therapy—shown to be safe and effective at reducing ischaemic complications including stroke following CABG. Aspirin 300mg first-line treatment of acute ischaemic stroke.
- Anticoagulation—should not be used routinely for treatment of acute stroke. If surgically indicated because of prosthetic valve, risk:benefit assessment with surgeon and neurologist.
- IV thrombolysis increasingly used in ischaemic stroke but contraindicated in context of recent surgery.
- Intra-arterial thrombolysis and mechanical clot disruption are under investigation for reperfusion in specific patients.
- Neurosurgical referral if:
  - Large middle cerebral artery infarction for consideration of decompressive craniectomy.
  - Primary intracranial haemorrhage with hydrocephalus.
- Supportive therapy:
  - Supplemental oxygen only if SaO$_2$ <95%.
  - BP—if hypertensive emergency (target <185/110mmHg).
  - Glycaemic control—hyperglycaemia associated with poor neurological outcome following both cardiac surgery and stroke. Blood glucose should be maintained 4–11mmol/L although no evidence that this improves outcome.
  - Temperature—hyperthermia should be avoided due to association with poor outcome following cardiac surgery and stroke.
  - Non-pharmacological DVT prophylaxis.
- Ongoing management of stroke should involve a specialist multi-disciplinary team who can address issues such as nutrition, physiotherapy, and secondary prevention.

Outcomes

- Several studies have shown an association with poor outcome and perioperative stroke in cardiac surgery. For example, following CABG stroke was associated with ↑ ICU stay, ↑ hospital stay, and ↑ hospital mortality (14.4% vs 2.7%).

Further reading

Hogue CW Jr, Palin CA, Arrowsmith JE. Cardiopulmonary bypass management and neurologic outcomes: an evidence-based appraisal of current practices. *Anesth Analg* 2006;103:21–37.

McKhann GM, Grega MA, Borowicz LM Jr, Baumgartner WA, Selnes OA. Stroke and encephalopathy after cardiac surgery: an update. *Stroke* 2006;37:562–71.

Stamou SC, Hill PC, Dangas G, Pfister AJ, Boyce SW, Dullum MK, *et al*. Stroke after coronary artery bypass: incidence, predictors, and clinical outcome. *Stroke* 2001;32:1508–13.

Immune system

Inflammatory response

Major surgery triggers a systemic inflammatory response. This is particularly so in cases involving CPB due to the exposure of the blood to the artificial surface. Biochemical and physiological signs of this response may be found in all post-cardiac surgery patients if one investigates carefully enough; however, it is clinically apparent in only a proportion and problematic in a minority. The systemic inflammatory response syndrome (SIRS) associated with major surgery is clinically indistinguishable from that triggered by infection (SIRS associated with infection is called sepsis).

Despite the avoidance of bypass a marked SIRS can still occur in off-pump patients as a result of the surgical trespass, cardiac manipulation, and circulatory disturbance.

Potential clinical features include:
- Vasodilation and subsequent hypotension
- Raised lactate
- Capillary leak (relative systemic hypovolaemia, impaired gas exchange, ↓ pulmonary compliance)
- Renal impairment
- ↑ susceptibility to infection
- Delirium.

Practice point

Fever, changes in white cell count, and rise in CRP are unreliable signs of infection immediately after cardiac surgery. Clinical history, the presence of other clinical signs (e.g. X-ray changes, sputum production), and culture results should be used in deciding whether to commence antimicrobial therapy in the first 48 hours postoperatively.

ARDS

Rarely, full blown ARDS ('pump lung') may occur as part of the inflammatory response after cardiac surgery. Treatment is supportive, as for ARDS from other causes.

Vasoplegia

Rarely, vasodilation associated with the SIRS triggered by cardiac surgery may be pronounced and intractable to normal therapy with alpha adrenergic agonists and vasopressin (severe vasoplegia). Nitric oxide is a powerful mediator of inflammatory vasodilation. Methylene blue inhibits nitric oxide-mediated vasodilation by a number of mechanisms (scavenges nitric oxide, inhibits nitric oxide synthetase and inhibits guanylate cyclase) and may be effective where other pressor agents are failing:

Dose regimen for methylene blue

In the presence of a good cardiac index, give a bolus of 1.5mg/kg (make up to 50mL with sterile water and infuse over 30 minutes). Response is rapid if it is going to occur. No major side effects are expected at this dose range. Urine and skin may become discoloured with the skin discolouration potentially interfering with pulse oximetry (but not oxygenation). The bolus may be followed by an infusion of 0.25–1.0mg/kg/hour for 6 hours starting 2 hours after the initial bolus.

Further reading

Faber P, Ronald A, Millar BW. Methythioninium chloride: pharmacology and clinical applications with special emphasis on nitric oxide mediated vasodilatory shock during cardiopulmonary bypass. *Anaesthesia* 2005;60: 575–87.

Heparin-induced thrombocytopenia

Heparin induced thrombocytopenia (HIT type 2) is an immunologically mediated condition where IGG antibodies are formed against heparin-platelet factor 4 (PF4) complexes. Heparin has a high affinity for PF4 and although neither is immunogenic by themselves antibodies are formed to the complexes. The antibodies cause pathological platelet activation and release of tissue factor (promotes thrombosis) from monocytes. HIT may be more likely when heparin exposure occurs in association with conditions that themselves increase the amount of circulating PF4, such as surgery and burns.

A non-immune HIT or HIT type 1 is also described. This is a benign self-limiting condition requiring no treatment. It is a result of the binding of heparin to PF4 per se. It is not associated with antibodies. It causes transient mild thrombocytopenia immediately within the first few days of heparin exposure due to platelet aggregation and sequestration.

The term HIT in common clinical usage refers to HIT type 2. HIT as discussed in this chapter refers to HIT type 2.

HIT is associated with thrombocytopenia but is a pro-thrombotic condition. It has a high mortality (30%) in its full clinical manifestation.

Incidence of HIT after exposure to unfractionated heparin has been estimated at between 1% and 5%, incidence is 5–10 times less than that after exposure to LMWH.

Platelet counts should be monitored regularly (usually daily) in all patients in cardiothoracic intensive care.

Clinical features

Thrombocytopenia
- Usually occurs 5–10 days after start of heparin therapy.
- Count usually increases within 4–14 days of stopping heparin.
- Count falls to 40,000–80,000 (<20,000 suggests alternate diagnosis).

Thrombosis
- Varies with clinical setting.
- Usually more common venous than arterial (4:1).
- Usually occurs after but may occur before thrombocytopenia.
- Includes DVT, PE, CVA, limb ischaemia, myocardial infarction and skin necrosis.
- May manifest as repeated circuit clotting in patient on haemofiltration.
- May occur after cessation of heparin therapy due to persistence of antibodies (antibodies usually disappear within 4 months).

HIT may be triggered by small amounts of heparin, e.g. in heparin flush used in central venous catheters or arterial lines.

Bleeding is uncommon in the absence of other causes of platelet dysfunction.

Diagnosis

Diagnosis is based on a combination of clinical signs and antibody detection.

Laboratory tests

Antibody assays are divided into those that test for platelet activation (functional assays) and other methods. Functional assays have a very high specificity (though still variable sensitivity) but are resource intensive and technically demanding. Most laboratories use other methods such as enzyme-linked immunoassays (ELISA) or particle gel immunoassay. These tests (particularly ELISA) are highly sensitive (close to 100%) and thus have a high negative predictive value, but are variably specific. Furthermore only a subset of antigens detected by these tests is functionally active in terms of platelet activation. They thus have a high false-positive rate (possibly in the order of 50% vs clinically significant HIT). Ideally, characterization requires detection with a high sensitivity test and characterization with a functional assay but this is will only be possible in laboratories with a special interest.

Practice point

Understand the type and significance of the HIT antibody tests used by your local laboratory.

Because of these difficulties a probabilistic approach must be taken. A formal scoring system such as the 4 Ts score can be incorporated into decision-making (Table 16.1).

Table 16.1 The 4 Ts scoring system

Category	Score		
	2	1	0
Degree of thrombocytopenia	>50% decrease or nadir 20–100 × 10⁹/L	30–50% decrease or nadir 10–19 × 10⁹/L	<30% decrease or nadir <10 × 10⁹/L
Timing of thrombocytopenia	5–10 days after exposure or <1 day if previous exposure within 1 month	>10 days after exposure or <1 day if previous exposure between 1 month and 1 year or unclear	No heparin in last year
Other causes of thrombocytopenia	None	Possible	Definite
Thrombotic phenomena/other clinical	Existing thrombosis, after heparin bolus, new skin necrosis or acute systemic reaction	Silent or recurrent thrombosis or erythematous skin lesions	None

Reproduced from Springer and Current Science, *Current Haematology Reports*, 2, 2, 2003, pp. 148–157, 'Laboratory diagnosis of immune heparin-induced thrombocytopenia', Warkentin TE, Heddle NM, with kind permission from Springer Science+Business Media B.V.

Score of 3 points or fewer gives a low risk of HIT and no further action is required. No laboratory tests are undertaken. Heparin does not need to be discontinued. Score of 6 points or more indicates a high risk of HIT. Score of 4 or 5 indicates an intermediate risk. If the score is 4 or over (intermediate- or high-risk patients) heparin should be discontinued, and antibody assay information sought. An alternative anticoagulation regimen should be started immediately as prophylaxis against thrombosis without waiting for laboratory results.

However, diagnosis is difficult as only a proportion of patients (5–30%) with antibodies develop thrombocytopenia. Only a proportion (30–70%) of patients with antibody-related thrombocytopenia develop thrombotic complications. Furthermore there are many causes of thrombocytopenia in critically ill patients. In a minority of patients with HIT (15%) thrombosis may occur with a normal platelet count. If there are pre-existing antibodies from a previous exposure the usual delay in onset may not occur ('rapid onset' HIT). Finally antibody detection varies depending on the method used and between laboratories. See Box 16.1.

> **Box 16.1 Differential diagnosis of thrombocytopenia**
>
> Many, but include:
> - Sepsis
> - Drug-induced
> - Haemofiltration
> - ECMO/VADS
> - CPB
> - Dilutional
> - Disseminated intravascular coagulation
> - Idiopathic thrombocytopenic purpura
> - PE
> - Liver disease
> - Hypersplenism
> - Malignancy
> - Immune disease (e.g. antiphospholipid syndrome, systemic lupus erythematosus)
> - (Very rarely) thrombotic thrombocytopenic purpura.

Management

Once HIT is diagnosed the principles of management are:
- Stop all heparin administration (including LMWHs and low-dose heparin flush)
- Start anticoagulation with an alternative parenteral anticoagulant.

See Table 16.2 for recommendations for cardiac surgery for patients with HIT.

Warfarin and other vitamin K antagonists in patients with HIT

Warfarin (and other vitamin K antagonists) are contraindicated in patients in the acute phase of HIT as initiation of warfarin therapy is associated with a procoagulant phase that lasts several days. Lower limb venous gangrene and severe skin necrosis have been described. In patients who are already on warfarin when they develop HIT, warfarin should be stopped and vitamin K should be administered.

Warfarin can be started once platelet count is >150 × 10⁹/L under cover of an alternative anticoagulant. Dosing should be cautious (5mg/day initially).

Platelet transfusion

It is unclear whether platelet transfusion actively precipitates thrombosis in HIT. Prophylactic platelet transfusion is unnecessary as bleeding is rare.

Alternative anticoagulants

This is an area which is currently evolving. All alternative strategies have balancing advantages and disadvantages. In patients without thrombosis the alternative anticoagulant should be continued until the platelet count has recovered to a stable plateau. Options include:

- Factor Xa antagonists:
  - Danaparoid—half-life of 24 hours with no specific antidote. Partially excreted in urine so accumulates in renal dysfunction. Monitor anti Xa level. Occasional (<10% cases) cross-reactivity with HIT IgG. Not available in USA.
  - Fondaparinux—synthetic heparin analogue. Forms anti PF4/heparin antibodies but these tend not to trigger HIT. Half-life of 18 hours. Renal excretion. No specific antidote.
- Direct thrombin inhibitors:
  - Short half-life. Generally given by IV infusion. No specific antidotes. Partly or largely excreted in urine so accumulate in renal failure.
- Lepirudin.
- Argatroban.
  - Hepatobiliary excretion. Contraindicated in liver cell failure. Monitor by APPT.
- Bivalirudin:
  - 80% cleared by enzymic proteolysis therefore advantageous in significant liver and kidney dysfunction. Requires dose adjustment in renal failure.

Table 16.2 Cardiac surgery for patients with HIT

Clinical picture	Immunological assay	Functional assay	Recommendation for surgery
Remote HIT	Negative	Negative	Use unfractionated heparin
Sub-acute HIT	Positive	Negative	Delay surgery until immune assay negative *Or:* use bivalirudin
Acute HIT	Positive	Positive	Delay surgery until both assays negative *Or:* use bivalirudin

Duration of treatment

Bilateral lower limb compression ultrasound should be performed in all patients with HIT whether or not there is clinical evidence of DVT. The presence of a DVT influences duration of anticoagulation.

- Patients with HIT and proven venous thrombosis (HITT) should be anticoagulated for 3–6 months.
- Patients with HIT without proven venous thrombosis (isolated HIT) have an elevated risk of thrombosis for at least 30 days. They should be anticoagulated for at least 1 month.

Further reading

Cuker A, Crowther MA. *Clinical Practice Guideline on the Evaluation and Management of Heparin-Induced Thrombocytopenia (HIT).* 2009. Available at: ℜ <http://www.hematology.org/Practice/Guidelines/2934.aspx>.

Linkins LA, Dans AL, Moores LK, Bona R, Davidson BL, Schulman S, et al. American College of Chest Physicians. Treatment and prevention of heparin-induced thrombocytopenia: Antithrombotic therapy and prevention of Thrombosis, 9th ed: American College of Chest Physicians Evidence-Based Clinical Practice Guidelines. *Chest* 2012;141(2 suppl):e4955–e5303.

Haematology

Coagulopathies

Cardiac surgery as a specialty is almost uniquely placed to provoke the development of coagulation abnormalities. There are numerous reasons why cardiac surgical patients may become coagulopathic.

Haemodilution

- Dilution of red cells occurs from addition of 1–1.5L of colloid/ crystalloid pump prime, the effect being exaggerated in patients with smaller blood volumes, i.e. low body weight.
- Haemodilution may also occur from volume replacement subsequent to haemorrhage or as treatment for postoperative hypotension.
- In addition, coagulation factors are also diluted—it is estimated that reductions to <30% of control levels are necessary before significant bleeding will occur although there is some individual variation. Factors V and VIII are most commonly reduced.

Haemorrhage

- Subsequent volume and red cell replacement may lead to the development of coagulopathy due to dilution, loss of factors, and loss of platelets.

Platelet damage

- Aside from dilution of platelets on bypass, mechanical damage from roller pumps or adsorption onto the membrane of the oxygenator may occur.
- Hypothermia-induced splenic sequestration of platelets has also been reported.

Antiplatelet therapy

- A significant number of cardiac patients are on antiplatelet medication prior to surgery.
- Most will be on aspirin alone, some will be on clopidogrel alone (or an alternative drug acting on the P2Y12 receptor), and some will be on both.
- Dual antiplatelet therapy is a significant concern with regard to perioperative bleeding and where safe to do so, most surgeons will stop clopidogrel 5 days in advance of surgery.
- Some emergency patients may also have been given glycoprotein IIb/ IIIa antagonists, e.g. tirofiban, which are very potent antiplatelet agents, acting as they do on the final common pathway of platelet activation.

Heparin–protamine mismatch

- There are numerous dosing regimens for administration of heparin for CPB and its subsequent reversal.
- It is important that heparin is adequately reversed at the end of the procedure.
- When the residual pump blood is administered to the patient towards the end of the case, some clinicians administer a further dose of protamine to cover any heparin present in that blood.

- In addition to a simple mismatch of heparin/protamine, the heparin–protamine complex may subsequently dissociate leading to the phenomenon of heparin rebound thus, in the presence of bleeding, coagulation tests including activated clotting time (ACT) should be repeated regularly.

Heparin-induced thrombocytopaenia

- This condition is, in fact, prothrombotic and is caused by platelet-activating antibodies which recognize complexes of platelet factor 4/ heparin.
- The platelet count typically falls between days 5 and 10 of heparin treatment and should be considered in all cases with decreasing platelet counts in the presence of heparin treatment.
- Treatment is withdrawal of heparin and substitution with another agent, e.g. danaparoid/bivalirudin.

Warfarinization

- In elective surgery, warfarin should be stopped several days in advance to allow the INR to return to normal (<1.5).
- Where a small residual effect exists, administration of a small dose of IV vitamin K (0.5–1mg) >12 hours prior to surgery should normalize the INR.
- For the emergency reversal of warfarin, the correct treatment is a prothrombin complex concentrate, e.g. Octaplex®, Beriplex®. Fresh frozen plasma (FFP) is not the treatment of choice.

Contact with artificial surfaces

- CPB acts to impair haemostasis; it activates fibrinolysis, impairs platelets as discussed, and affects coagulation factors.
- The extracorporeal circuit contains a large surface of thrombogenic material; activation of thrombin results in fibrinolytic activity, activation of complement, and inflammatory mediators.
- Denaturation of plasma proteins/factors may occur at blood–air interfaces, a common situation in cardiac surgery.

Temperature

- Patients are often cooled during bypass and may remain mildly/moderately hypothermic on return to the ITU impacting on normal coagulation.

Blood conservation

From what has already been discussed, it can be no surprise that cardiac surgery is a high blood-using specialty, estimated to use 15% of the UK blood supply. While the blood supply could be considered to be the safest it has ever been there are still recognizable risks associated with transfusion of red cells and blood products.

SHOT (Serious Hazards of Transfusion) reports annually on adverse events associated with transfusion:

- Incorrect component transfusion accounts for 25% of reports
- Acute and haemolytic transfusion reactions account for 31%
- Transfusion-related acute lung injury accounts for 2%
- Transfusion-transmitted infections 0.6%
- The risk of variant Creutzfeldt–Jakob disease is, as yet, unknown.

In addition, several large retrospective studies have demonstrated an association between transfusion and long- and short-term increases in mortality even if only 1 unit of red cells has been transfused.

Blood is also an expensive and finite resource. These facts considered, it is appropriate that attempts are made to decrease our use of red cells and blood products and to use the resource appropriately.

Blood conservation could be considered to address three specific areas:

- Increasing or optimizing patients' haemoglobin preoperatively
- Decreasing blood loss intra- and postoperatively
- Optimizing transfusion practice using the best available evidence.

Increasing preoperative haemoglobin

Anaemia

- Anaemia is an independent predictor of mortality in the cardiac surgical population.
- It has been demonstrated that up to a quarter of patients presenting for cardiac surgery have ↓ iron stores. These patients have lower admission Hb, receive more red cells during their hospital stay, and have lower discharge Hb than their normal counterparts. However screening patients far enough in advance for treatment to be useful presents logistical problems for most units.
- Oral iron salts should increase Hb by 1g/dL every 10 days and, although usually well tolerated, treatment should last for at least 4–6 weeks to allow for an increase in Hb.
- IV iron has been associated with allergic reactions so is not without risk compared to oral formulations.
- Erythropoietin is not currently approved in the UK for preoperatively increasing Hb (except in Jehovah's Witnesses).

Autologous transfusion

Most Health Boards do offer autologous transfusion, however cardiac disease is a contraindication.

Decreasing blood loss intra- and postoperatively

There are several possible points of intervention:

Acute normovolaemic haemodilution

The principle behind this technique is that:

- After induction in suitable patients (e.g. Hb >12g/dL), a volume of blood (e.g. 5mL/kg) can be removed from the patient and stored for re-infusion at the end of surgery.
- The volume removed is replaced with colloid to maintain normovolaemia.
- The advantages of this technique are that it is fairly simple, relatively inexpensive, and means that blood lost intraoperatively is of a lower haematocrit, therefore fewer red cells are lost.
- The blood transfused at the end of the procedure will raise the haematocrit and Hb and also contains platelets which function as well as they did preoperatively.

Pharmaceutical interventions

Antifibrinolytic agents

- Tranexamic acid:
  - A lysine analogue which binds to the lysine binding site of the plasminogen molecule displacing it from fibrin.
  - It has been proven to decrease blood loss, decrease transfusion, and to decrease the frequency of surgical re-exploration.
  - Having largely replaced aprotinin in cardiac practice, several recent studies have suggested that its use may be associated with similar complications.
- Aprotinin:
  - Aprotinin's licence has been withdrawn, however, some centres continue to use it for high-risk patients off-licence on a named-patient only basis.

DDAVP®

- A synthetic vasopressin derivative which acts by recruitment of von Willebrand factor thus increasing platelet adhesion.
- It also increases concentrations of factor VIII and tissue plasminogen activator.
- It is not commonly used in the UK and good evidence of benefit is slim.

NovoSeven®

Recombinant factor VIIa has been used in an attempt to arrest catastrophic haemorrhage in extremis:

- It has been reported that there is a significant increase in thrombotic events in those treated outside its licensed indications for haemophilia and its use has accordingly become controversial.
- Its use therefore is at the discretion of the attending medical staff in discussion with haematologists.

Cell salvage

- Evidence supports the use of intraoperative cell salvage in cardiac surgery.
- However, there is a requirement for significant financial investment in terms of machine purchase, machine maintenance, purchase of disposables, and training of staff.

- Given the cost of 1 unit of red cells may be quoted as £150, cell salvage offers potentially significant savings.
- Blood lost from the surgical field is washed to remove contaminants, debris, heparin, cytokines, etc. and is resuspended in normal saline for reinfusion.
- Most systems concentrate the blood to a haematocrit of at least 60%.
- This blood, however, will contain no coagulation factors or platelets.
- A postoperative system which acts as a mediastinal drain is also offered by Haemonetics (cardioPAT®) and has proved useful in our practice.
- It is important to note that some Jehovah's Witness patients may accept cell salvage as part of their treatment.

Decreasing haemodilution by pump prime

Moving the machine as close as possible to the patient and cutting arterial and venous lines to an appropriate length can decrease the amount of volume added at the time of bypass and hence decrease haemodilution.

Mini bypass

This is a relatively new technique which is used in few units and is somewhat more than simple miniaturization of a traditional bypass circuit requiring specific training for the perfusionists.

However, its aim is to minimize the inflammatory response to bypass which is done in several ways:

- Haemodilution is ↓ (may be able to reduce prime to as little as 150mL).
- Minimizes the surface area of the circuit and oxygenator.
- *Lower suction is applied to the venous side of the circulation than in conventional bypass, decreasing damage to blood cells.*
- The centrifugal pump is also less damaging to red cells and platelets.
- There is no blood–air interface as there is no venous reservoir.
  Accordingly:
  - Blood loss is ↓.
  - Transfusion is ↓.
- May decrease myocardial injury and postoperative dysrhythmias.
- May minimize renal and intestinal injury.

There have, however, been significant concerns regarding the risk of air embolism.

Use of topical haemostatic agents

Use of these agents has also been suggested:

- Employing localized compression as a scaffold for clot formation, e.g. surgicel or
- As anastomotic sealants as a spray.
- There seems to be some evidence of ↓ bleeding but limited evidence of ↓ transfusion requirements.

Topical antifibrinolytics

There is some evidence of a benefit of administration of antifibrinolytic agents such as tranexamic acid directly to the wound at closure.

Off-pump procedures

These may confer advantages (OPCAB) by avoiding some of the potential provoking factors of bypass (haemodilution, contact with artificial surfaces, platelet damage).

Avoid excesses of blood pressure

Hypertension may lead to ↑ blood loss from suture lines after aortotomy.

Good surgical haemostasis

Never to be underestimated in reducing blood loss.

Optimizing transfusion practice

MSBOS (maximum surgical blood ordering schedule)

Unit-specific protocols for ordering a predetermined number of units of blood for each surgical procedure based on likelihood of use have been proven to decrease blood wastage. Good practice states that the cross-match to transfusion ratio should be no greater than 2:1.

Guidelines/transfusion triggers

There are several different guidelines available to optimize transfusion practice, some looking specifically at cardiac surgery.

Recent STS/ SCA guidelines suggests:

- Adoption of a transfusion trigger of 7g/dL Hb postoperatively although each patient should be assessed individually for evidence of impaired oxygen delivery.
- There is no evidence supporting transfusion where Hb >10g/dL.
- A trigger of 6g/dL is suggested during bypass.
- Given that a significant volume of colloid has been added during bypass, it is normal to tolerate lower Hb concentrations in the expectation that the patient will increase their urine output and the haematocrit will rise over the first few hours post bypass.

Algorithms

Introduction of a transfusion algorithm alone has been proven to decrease transfusion requirements. These should, of course, be evidence-based.

Near-patient testing

This will be discussed further (see 📖 Viscoelastic tests, p. 165) however there are several cardiac surgical publications demonstrating ↓ red cell and blood product use with ROTEM®/TEG® and publications which also demonstrate significant cost savings.

Individually the effect of many of these interventions is small. It is only through the adoption of a multimodal and multidisciplinary approach to blood conservation that the best results can be obtained.

Point-of-care testing

Point-of-care testing may be defined as any analytical test performed by a healthcare professional outside the laboratory setting which should generate results comparable to the local laboratory with matching reference ranges. Unfortunately laboratory testing can be slow and results will reflect the patient's status at the time the samples were taken; in cardiac surgery the situation may have altered significantly by the time the results are reported. The aim with all point-of-care tests is to obtain results more quickly than could be obtained by regular laboratory testing, that they may more appropriately guide therapy.

Blood gas analysis

Will give rapid and reliable information on:
- Hb concentrations and haematocrits to guide transfusion decisions
- Electrolyte disturbances (with particular reference to K and Ca)
- Acid–base abnormalities and lactate concentrations
- Glucose.

Haemoglobin analysers

Most units would use blood gas analysis for Hb measurement nowadays; however, analysers such as HemoCue® are available for assessment of Hb.

Coagulation monitors

Hand-held monitors of coagulation are available giving prothrombin time (PT) and INR results.

ACT

Although the ACT is a fairly crude test (using a tube containing an activator such as diatomaceous earth and a magnet rotating in a well) it is commonly used in cardiac units as a means of monitoring the effect of heparin administration.
- There are several devices available some offering heparinase-adjusted results, some offering accelerated results.
- Unit protocols dictate the acceptable levels for commencement of CPB but 400 or 480 seconds are common.
- It is important to note that the ACT is not solely dependent on the effects of heparin; it also depends on platelet and fibrinogen interactions.
- *After protamine administration, a further test is performed to assess a return towards baseline.*

Hepcon®

An automated device which measures:
- The heparin dose response
- Heparin–protamine titration, predicting the required dose of protamine
- Some authors have suggested such direct measurements of heparin concentration as a more appropriate measurement and as a better method to monitor anticoagulation on bypass and heparin reversal.

Viscoelastic tests

These tests were first described in the 1940s and have regained favour in the last 15 years as concerted attempts have been made to decrease blood transfusion.

- There are two commercially available systems—ROTEM® and TEG®.
- Both are viscoelastic tests, i.e. they test the 'stickiness' of clot and provide an overview of the coagulation system including assessment of platelet function and of the plasma-based factors.
- They test not only how rapidly clot forms but if the clot becomes and remains stable.
- The systems both rely on placing blood in a cuvette into which a pin is inserted. In ROTEM® this pin rotates back and forth by approximately 4° (Fig. 17.1) and in TEG the cup rotates by a similar amount. As clot forms between the pin and the wall of the cup, this change in tension is detected and is transformed into the ROTEM®/TEG® trace (Fig. 17.2).
- The traces produced are somewhat similar and each parameter can be related to certain aspects of the coagulation process allowing a rapid and accurate diagnosis of any coagulopathy and therefore the institution of early appropriate treatment.
- CT (clotting time)/r time = the time from the start of the test until the first clot forms—prolonged by factor deficiency and heparin excess. Performance of a HEPTEM/heparinase test would help differentiate.
- CFT (clot formation time)/k time = the time from clot first forming until the amplitude reaches 20mm—prolonged by factor deficiency or platelet abnormality.
- Alpha angle reflects rate of clot formation.
- MCF (maximum clot firmness) reflects deficiencies of fibrin or platelet function abnormality. Performance of a FIBTEM test would help differentiate.
- MA (maximum amplitude) is the equivalent of MCF for TEG® and is said to reflect platelet abnormality although functional fibrinogen testing is available for TEG®.
- ML (maximum lysis) reflects fibrinolysis.
- It has been suggested that these tests are the gold standard in diagnosing hyperfibrinolysis.

There are various tests available for both machines. ROTEM® specifically uses the addition of different activating agents to further localize any abnormality as part of the diagnostic algorithm:

- It is important to recognize that neither system will identify the effects of drugs (antiplatelet agents, warfarin) on routine testing.
- While it is important to rapidly identify the presence of coagulopathy, it is equally important to identify the absence of a coagulopathy which would imply a surgical cause for any haemorrhage allowing early re-exploration.

Use of thromboelastometry or thromboelastography has been recommended by QIS (Quality Improvement Scotland) as a clinical and cost-effective measure in cardiac surgery.

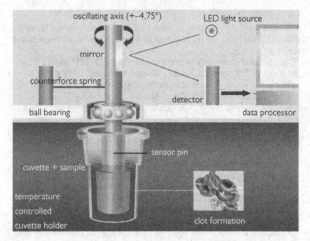

Figure 17.1 The ROTEM® mechanism of action. With kind permission from Tem International GmbH <http://www.rotem.de/site/index.php?option=com_content& view=article&id=1&Itemid=7&lang=en>.

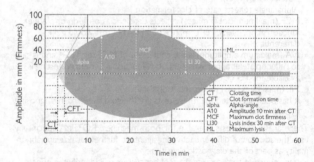

Figure 17.2 A ROTEM® trace. With kind permission from Tem International GmbH <http://www.rotem.de/site/index.php?option=com_content&view=article&id=1& Itemid=7&lang=en>.

Platelet function tests

Given the increasing use of antiplatelet agents either alone or in combination, platelet function testing may be an increasingly useful/valuable diagnostic tool:

- There are several devices commercially available, e.g. Multiplate®, VerifyNow®, PFA-100®.
- While each use different technologies to obtain the results, they will all give information on platelet function and most give information on the effects of antiplatelet agents.
- While resistance to aspirin is rare, responsiveness to clopidogrel varies between studies but resistance may be as high as 40%. Those who are not responsive are clearly no more likely to bleed than those not on the drug.
- These tests may allow patients at genuinely ↑ risk of bleeding perioperatively to be targeted by some of the more expensive blood conservation strategies.

Specific patient groups

The thoracic patient

Routine care of the thoracic patient

Thoracic surgery in adults includes surgery to the lungs (including lung transplantation), pleura, thymus, oesophagus, and other thoracic structures as well as the chest wall. Thoracic procedures include lobar resection, pneumonectomy for malignant and non-malignant conditions, mediastinoscopy and mediastinotomy, and bronchoscopy for diagnostic and interventional indications. Video-assisted thoracoscopic surgery (VATS) is performed for drainage and investigation of effusions, lung resection, sympathectomy, and removal of mediastinal tumours. Other procedures include the surgical management of air-leaks, management of empyema, operations on the chest wall, endobronchial laser surgery, and tracheal stenting and oesophagectomy. All of these patient groups may require admission to cardiothoracic ICU.

The routine care of thoracic surgical patients is aimed at promoting rapid recovery and reducing complications. Thoracotomy is a major operation and is one of the most painful. The nature of the surgery and the common comorbidities of this patient group such as respiratory disease result in an ↑ incidence of respiratory complications. Patients may be admitted to critical care for routine postoperative care in level 2 beds or for level 3 care as a result of a complication of surgery, whether immediately postoperatively such as bleeding or as a later complication such as respiratory failure.

Routine postoperative care

Analgesia

Pain is the enemy of recovery and will prevent adequate coughing and deep breathing. After lung resection, the patient will generally have a regional technique *in situ* such as paravertebral blockade or thoracic epidural analgesia. This is usually part of a balanced analgesic technique with the administration of regular paracetamol and non-steroidal analgesics. Patient-controlled analgesia is often used to supplement analgesic efficacy of paravertebral block.

Oxygen therapy

Oxygen therapy should be given to overcome the V/Q mismatch associated with thoracic surgery. Generally humidified oxygen is administered to avoid the drying effects on secretions of the pipeline gases. Oxygen should be prescribed to achieve a SpO_2 of 94–98% or 88–92% in patients with chronic obstructive pulmonary disease (COPD) at risk of hypercapnic respiratory failure. High oxygen concentrations may promote absorption atelectasis and lung injury and may also be dangerous in COPD patients with hypoxia-dependant respiratory drive.

Chest drainage

Intercostal chest drains are inserted at the end of thoracic surgery to allow drainage of blood (basal drain) and air (apical drain) from the damaged lung. Typically these are each connected to an underwater drainage bottle which operates as a one-way valve which is set at $2cmH_2O$. An additional bottle may be added to allow low pressure suction to be applied to encourage lung expansion. Low-level suction at $20cmH_2O$ can be applied. Continued air leak is evidenced by bubbling of the drains.

The pleural drain should swing with respiration if it is patent and bubbling indicates air leak from damage lung and if severe may suggest bronchopleural fistula.

Automated portable drain systems are now available which are battery driven and generate a constant negative pressure and display a digital display of the air leak in mL/minute.

Physiotherapy and mobilization

Physiotherapy and early mobilization are essential for the thoracic patient. The thoracic patient should be managed sitting up at all times. On day 1 they should be mobilized to a chair and begin weight bearing as soon as possible.

Some patients who are at risk of atelectasis and hypoxemia in the postoperative period should have CPAP or BIPAP as preventive measures.

Minitracheostomy

When the there is concern that a patient may be unable to cough adequately due to weakness, laryngeal nerve palsy, or excessive secretions, some units will consider the use of a minitracheostomy to assist secretion clearance.

Venous thromboembolism prophylaxis

All thoracic patients should have venous thromboembolism (VTE) prophylaxis usually in the form of LMWH commenced preoperatively. Epidural catheters should not be inserted or removed within 12 hours of the administration of LMWH. The timing of LMWH should allow preoperative epidural catheter insertion. We give LMWH at 6pm the night before surgery and every 24 hours thereafter.

Fluid administration

It is generally accepted that thoracic patient should be relatively fluid restricted and fluids should be prescribed with caution. A typical post-op prescription would be 1mL/kg/hour of Hartmann's solution up to a maximum of 70mL/hour. There is an association between post thoracotomy ALI and excessive fluid administration; however, the causal relationship has never been conclusively demonstrated. Units will have local policies for fluid administration.

Antibiotic prophylaxis

Antibiotics are commonly administered after thoracotomy for 24 hours. Local protocols should be followed.

Bronchodilators

In asthmatics and patients with reversibility of their airways disease, bronchodilators are indicated. Generally the routine inhalers are continued through the perioperative period although inhalers may be converted to nebulizers. Salbutamol may contribute to the risk of postoperative atrial fibrillation and as such should not be routinely prescribed. Ipratropium is better tolerated and can be used where the benefits of β_2 agonists are borderline.

Nutrition

Nutritional deficiencies are common in thoracic patients as a consequence of chronic infection (empyema), cancer cachexia, and dysphagia (oesophageal disorders). Early feeding is encouraged and where appetite is poor and/or dysphagia prevents consumption of adequate calories enteral feeding should be established.

Postoperative respiratory failure

Respiratory complications occur in 25% of patients after lung resection. Of these, the more severe will require admission to ICU and up to 5% may require positive pressure ventilation. The reasons for postoperative respiratory failure are multifold. Patients may have significant underlying respiratory disease and then may fail to tolerate the loss of lung function associated with the lung resection. Recovery from surgery is complicated by postoperative pain and its consequences, such as the restriction in coughing and deep breathing. Opiate analgesia may also suppress cough reflexes, and cause sedation and hypoventilation. These variables conspire to cause atelectasis and sputum retention which may develop into postoperative pneumonia. ALI after lung resection is a major contributing factor in many patients and may be underdiagnosed.

Aetiology of postoperative respiratory failure

- Atelectasis
- ALI/ARDS
- Pneumonia
- Severe underlying respiratory disease
- Excessive resection
- PE
- Aspiration.

Thoracic conditions which may result in respiratory failure

- Blunt chest trauma and lung contusion
- Chest stabbing
- Bronchopleural fistula
- Empyema.

Principles of management

When respiratory failure occurs after thoracic surgery, the causes are often multifactorial and treatment is both supportive and aimed at the underlying causes. Nosocomial respiratory infection may accompany atelectasis and ALI. Non-invasive ventilation reduces the requirement for intubation and intermittent positive pressure ventilation (IPPV) and improves outcomes in type 2 respiratory failure. The following interventions may be indicated:
- Non-invasive ventilation:
  - Nasal CPAP
  - BiPAP
  - CPAP and pressure support
  - Hood CPAP
- Minitracheostomy
- Intubation and IPPV
- Early tracheostomy
- Physiotherapy and mobilization
- Sputum culture and antibiotics:
  - Hospital acquired vs community acquired
- Fluid restriction

- Bronchodilators:
  - Beta agonists: salbutamol
  - Cholinergic: ipratropium
  - Steroids: beclometasone
- Systemic steroids
- Enteral feeding
- DVT prophylaxis.

Post-thoracotomy acute lung injury

Formerly known as post-pneumonectomy pulmonary oedema but also occurs after lesser resections. Often rapidly progressive syndrome of non-cardiogenic pulmonary infiltration and hypoxia developing after thoracotomy. Clinical, radiological, and histopathological characteristics are similar to ARDS. A bimodal distribution of onset has been described.

Definition

ALI/ARDS diagnosed as per the American-European consensus definition:
- Acute onset of hypoxaemia: PaO_2/FiO_2 ratio <300mmHg for ALI/<200mmHg for ARDS (regardless of level of PEEP).
- Bilateral infiltrates on CXR.
- PAWP <18mmHg (but rarely measured in this group) or no evidence of left atrial hypertension.

Incidence
- Reports vary: 2–5% after lobectomy, 2.5–15% after pneumonectomy.

Outcome
- Mortality 40–60%. Some series report 100% for ARDS requiring intubation.

Early or 'primary' ALI
- Postoperative days 0–3.

Pathophysiology
Both ipsilateral and contralateral lungs are exposed to inflammatory and oxidative insults secondary to:
- Ipsilateral: atelectasis, surgical manipulation, ischaemia-reperfusion
- Contralateral: hyperoxia, high airway pressures (barotrauma), hyperinflation (volutrauma), hyperperfusion.

Risk factors
- High intraoperative ventilatory pressures (both duration of one lung ventilation and peak airway pressure appear to be important)
- Large tidal volumes on one-lung ventilation
- Excessive IV volume replacement
- Pneumonectomy > lobectomy > lesser resections
- Right sided resection > left
- Preoperative alcohol abuse
- Preoperative respiratory function (forced expiratory volume in 1 second (FEV_1)).

Late or 'secondary' ALI
- Post-operative days 3–10
- Secondary to obvious causes:
  - Pneumonia
  - Aspiration
  - Bronchopulmonary fistula.

Prevention

Prevention is key. Early use of non-invasive ventilation is favoured to avoid intubation. Mortality increases dramatically if positive pressure ventilation is required.

- Lung protective ventilatory strategies during one-lung ventilation are widely believed to be of benefit (limited evidence base):
  - Reduced FiO_2: 30–50% in absence of hypoxia
  - Low physiological tidal volume ~6mL/kg or less
  - Pressure-limited ventilation—minimize peak pressure
  - Prevention of atelectasis through use of PEEP ~5cmH₂O
  - Use of recruitment manoeuvres
- Fluid restriction:
  - Minimize IVI—restrictive/goal-directed approach intraoperatively and for following 24–48 hours
  - Use of vasopressors to treat (non-haemorrhagic) hypotension (e.g. noradrenaline 0.02–0.2mcg/kg/min)
- Inhaled β2 agonists (e.g. nebulized salbutamol 2.5–5mg 4-hourly)
- Chest physiotherapy, early mobilization
- Early use of non-invasive ventilation in at-risk patient.

Management

It is essential to identify and treat any underlying primary cause for respiratory failure, e.g. aspiration, pneumonia, pneumothorax, PE:

- Oxygen
- Chest physiotherapy
- Close attention to fluid balance:
  - Consider induced diuresis
  - Use of vasopressors to treat (non-haemorrhagic) hypotension (e.g. noradrenaline 0.02–0.2mcg/kg/min)
- Non-invasive ventilation
- Intubation and positive pressure ventilation:
  - Lung protective ventilation with limited tidal volumes and minimizing airway pressures (see Chapter 26)
- Experimental/proposed therapies described in the literature (predominantly observational data in small numbers of patients):
  - Corticosteroids
  - Inhaled nitric oxide
  - Extracorporeal CO_2 removal.

Further reading

Licker M, de Perrot M, Spiliopoulos A, Robert J, Diaper J, Chevalley C, et al. Risk factors for acute lung injury after thoracic surgery. *Anesth Analg* 2003;97:1558–65.

Chest drainage

The intrapleural drain is essential for treatment and prevention of pneumothorax and drainage of pleural collections of blood, pleural effusion, or empyema. They are routinely sited after thoracotomy and lung resection. Classically two drains are inserted: an apical drain for air drainage and a basal drain for drainage of blood. Single drains placed apically with basal sideholes are now popular and cause less pain.

After cardiac surgery, mediastinal and pleural drains are inserted for drainage of blood.

Insertion of intercostal drains can be dangerous particularly when there are pleural adhesions. Special care should be taken when there has been previous intrathoracic surgery.

Full aseptic technique should be used and the drain position should be confirmed on CXR afterwards.

Drains *in situ* should never be advanced further into chest as this can introduce infection.

Indications for chest drain insertion

- Pneumothorax in any ventilated patient
- Tension pneumothorax after initial needle decompression
- Persistent or recurrent pneumothorax after simple aspiration
- Large secondary spontaneous pneumothorax in patients >50 years
- Malignant pleural effusion
- Empyema and complicated parapneumonic pleural effusion
- Traumatic haemopneumothorax
- Postoperative, e.g. thoracotomy, oesophagectomy, cardiac surgery.

Pre-insertion check

- Consent.
- Bleeding risk: check coagulation screen and platelets if risk of abnormality.
- Diagnostic challenges: it is important to differentiate between the presence of collapse and a pleural effusion when the chest radiograph shows a unilateral 'whiteout'. Ultrasound can be useful.
- Lung densely adherent to the chest wall throughout the hemithorax is an absolute contraindication to chest drain insertion.
- The drainage of a post-pneumonectomy space should only be carried out by or after consultation with a thoracic surgeon.

Potential complications

- Bleeding
- Damage to underlying lung
- Cardiac damage with trochar
- Hepatic or splenic injury
- Injury to intercostal neurovascular bundle
- Infection of intrapleural space and sepsis.

Drainage arrangements

See Figs 18.1, 18.2, and 18.3.

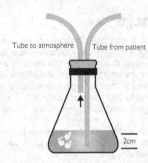

Figure 18.1 An underwater seal for pneumothorax. Courtesy of Atrium, Maquet Getinge Group.

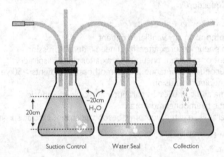

Figure 18.2 An underwater seal combined with drainage bottle and suction bottle. Courtesy of Atrium, Maquet Getinge Group.

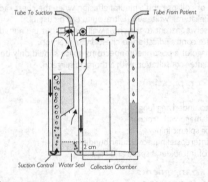

Figure 18.3 An example of a modern drainage system which allows underwater seal, drainage of blood or fluids, and the application of controlled suction in one sealed unit. Courtesy of Atrium, Maquet Getinge Group.

Chest drainage techniques

- Chest drainage is a dangerous procedure and should be only be performed by trained individuals.
- Bedside ultrasound reduces the risk of intercostal chest drain (ICD) insertion.
- A Seldinger technique for introduction of small-bore ICD (8–14FG) may reduce risks of damage to the underlying lung and is used for pleural fluid aspiration.
- A large-bore (>24FG) size of ICD tube must be inserted when blood drainage is required.
- The insertion site should be in the 'triangle of safety' (see Fig. 18.4). This is the triangle bordered by the anterior border of the latissimus dorsi, the lateral border of the pectoralis major muscle, a line superior to the horizontal level of the nipple, and an apex below the axilla.

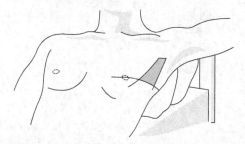

Figure 18.4 Diagram to illustrate the 'safe triangle'. Reproduced from *Thorax*, D. Laws, et al., BTS guidelines for the insertion of a chest drain, 58, Suppl 2, pp. 53–59, copyright 2003, with permission from BMJ Publishing Group Ltd and British Thoracic Society.

Removal of drains

- Drains for pneumothorax are generally not removed until bubbling has stopped and CXR shows lung re-expansion.
- When bleeding has become insignificant.
- There is no benefit in clamping the chest drain before removal.
- CXR should be repeated after drain removal.

Thoracic surgical drainage system

- Suction of 10–20cmH$_2$O can be applied if the is lung not fully inflated by attaching an additional underwater drain bottle and attaching to wall with low pressure suction.

Electronic drainage systems

Electronic systems driven by battery and/or mains have potential benefits for thoracic surgery. The pump applies continuous suction and is small and has no fluid level which allows easier patient mobility. The pump applies a constant level of suction and gives a digital display of air leak in mL/minute. This allows better quantification of air leak and the drains can generally be removed when the air leak falls below 50mL/hour.

Mobile pleural drainage

When patients with intrapleural drains are transferred a flutter valve (or Heimlich valve) can be used if there is air leak without significant fluid or blood drainage.

Further reading

Laws D, Neville E, Duffy J; Pleural Diseases Group, Standards of Care Committee, British Thoracic Society. BTS guidelines for the insertion of a chest drain. *Thorax* 2003;58(suppl 2):ii53–ii59.

Bronchopleural fistula

A bronchopleural fistula (BPF) is a persistent communication between the bronchial tree and the pleural space. Patients with bronchopleural fistula present particular management challenges. The BPF results in an air leak from the lung and consequently there is acquired infection of the pleural space and empyema. Initial treatment often involves drainage of the pleural space which can be difficult as there is often loculation of the empyema. The chronic infection in the pleural space progressively results in debility and weight loss. Spillage of infected pleural fluid into the airway contaminates the good lung and results in recurrent chest infection.

Causes of BPF

- Post-pneumonectomy stump dehiscence
- Carcinoma of lung
- Tuberculosis
- Traumatic.

Management

In the event of a patient with BPF requiring intubation and ventilation, special consideration should be given to the risk of inadequate ventilation due to massive air leak and airway contamination. If the BPF is post pneumonectomy, lung isolation may be required and the placement of a double-lumen tube may be necessary. A rapid sequence induction with pre-oxygenation and accurate placement of a double-lumen tube with the help of a fibrescope is the technique of choice. Alternative ventilation strategies such as the use of jet ventilation or high-frequency oscillation may have a place when the air leak is persistent and severe. These techniques are not universally available.

The surgical management of the BPF will be guided by the thoracic surgical team.

Thoracic airway obstruction

Thoracic patients with life-threatening obstruction to their trachea and lower airways may be admitted to cardiothoracic ICU for emergency management. After initial stabilization, investigations and diagnosis lead to definitive treatment.

Aetiology of airway obstruction

- Foreign body
- Trauma (post intubation, burns, and other forms of trauma)
- Neoplasm of the trachea or major bronchus
- Mediastinal lymphoma
- Thymic tumours.

Diagnostic investigations often include CT scan, rigid bronchoscopy, and mediastinoscopy with biopsy for histological diagnosis. Relief of airway obstruction may require initial intubation and treatment with steroids and/ or radiological placement of airway stents prior to definitive treatment with further surgery or chemotherapy/radiotherapy.

Lung volume reduction surgery

Conventional lung volume reduction surgery (LVRS) is a palliative operation in patients with severe emphysema. The surgical removal of emphysematous lung areas reduces the hyperexpanded lung volume and gives mechanical advantage. This may result in improvement in life expectancy and symptoms. Lesser forms of surgery such as simple bullectomy may also be performed in emphysematous patients. A major study of LVRS showed that overall, LVRS increases the chance of improved exercise capacity but does not confer a survival advantage over medical therapy. It does yield a survival advantage for patients with both predominantly upper-lobe emphysema and low baseline exercise capacity. Patients previously reported to be at high risk and those with non-upper-lobe emphysema and high baseline exercise capacity were poor candidates for LVRS, because of ↑ mortality and negligible functional gain.

LVRS can be performed by various surgical approaches such as VATs, minithoracotomy, thoracotomy, or sternotomy. These may be unilateral or bilateral, or staged bilateral.

The major complications seen are respiratory failure often complicated by persistent air leaks from staple lines in the poor quality lungs. The requirement for positive pressure ventilation carries a very high morbidity and mortality.

Further reading

Fishman A, Martinez F, Naunheim K, Piantadosi S, Wise R, Ries A, et al. A randomized trial comparing lung-volume-reduction surgery with medical therapy for severe emphysema. NEJM 2003;348(21):2059–73.

Lung volume reduction surgery

The adult patient with congenital heart disease

Introduction

The success of paediatric cardiac services has resulted in a significant growth in the population of adults with congenital heart disease (ACHD):

- In Westernized societies the number of adults with congenital heart disease is now greater than the number of children.
- Survival to adulthood is now estimated to be ~90%.
- The majority of adults with ACHD have a good quality of life with families to support and jobs to maintain.

The spectrum of anatomies comprising ACHD is wide, ranging from simple lesions such as patent ductus arteriosus to complex single ventricle morphologies. The anatomy, however, is only part of the condition. The more challenging aspect in the care of these patients is appreciation of the resultant physiology. A 'simple' patent ductus arteriosus may manifest in the adult as Eisenmenger syndrome with pulmonary hypertension.

Patients with ACHD may present to CICU in three circumstances:

Postoperatively following cardiac intervention

Very few congenital cardiac procedures are curative. Adults may require cardiac intervention (surgical or transcatheter) in several circumstances:

- Primary repair of anatomy
- Repair of sequelae of primary anatomical repair
- Intervention for unrelated problem, e.g. CABG
- Cardiac and/or pulmonary transplantation.

Postoperatively following non-cardiac surgery

Patients with complex ACHD benefit from perioperative CICU care for non-cardiac surgical procedures, including obstetric interventions. The specialist's appreciation of the physiological balance optimizes the ICU outcome.

Management of medical emergency

Medical emergencies may critically destabilize a patient with ACHD; for example, acute severe pneumonia in a single ventricular physiology. These patients also benefit from CICU care although the limited evidence base suggests that despite this specialist care the outcome for these patients is often poor.

The additional consideration for patients with ACHD is that their cardiac history may be only part of their condition. There are a wide range of syndromes that include cardiac defects. These syndromes need to be understood to fully appreciate a patient's needs. Some patients with ACHD have learning difficulties that significantly impacts communication.

Key point

For all patients with ACHD contact their base clinical team (cardiology/GP) to ensure that the CICU team have a full understanding of the anatomy, physiology, and comorbidities.

ACHD has many eponymous syndromes and operations. This confounds the understanding of specific lesions and interventions. Some of the more common terms are described in Table 19.1.

Table 19.1 List of more common terms and descriptions of lesions and interventions

Term	Description
ALCAPA	*Anomalous left coronary artery from pulmonary artery*: usually presents and repaired in childhood, but may cause left ventricular systolic dysfunction
ASD	*Atrial septal defect*: most commonly *secundum* and potentially repairable with transcatheter device, *primum* defects also called partial atrioventricular defect, *superior sinus venosus* defects are associated with partial anomalous pulmonary venous drainage, uncommon defects include inferior sinus venosus defects and coronary sinus defects
AVSD	*Atrioventricular septal defect*: these may be partial affecting either the atrial septum or ventricular septum, or complete with a resultant common atrioventricular valve
Balanced circulation	Pulmonary blood supply arises from the systemic arterial circulation. The balance of systemic and pulmonary flow is critical. Systemic vasodilation (e.g. anaesthetic agents) reduces pulmonary blood flow. Pulmonary vasoconstriction reduces pulmonary blood flow increasing cyanosis. Systemic vaodilatation can be countered with systemic vasoconstriction, e.g. with phenylephrine
Blalock–Taussig shunt	Palliative shunt connecting the subclavian artery to the ipsilateral PA, to increase pulmonary blood flow. Classical shunt transected the subclavian artery to fashion an end-to-side anastomosis with the PA. Modified shunts use a synthetic interposition tube graft. Operation achieved through thoracotomy. Blood pressure may be falsely low in the ipsilateral arm
Concordance	Connection of two structures on the same side morphologically—right atrium to right ventricle
Congenitally corrected transposition of the great arteries (ccTGA; Fig. 19.3)	Atrioventricular and ventriculo-arterial discordance (double discordance): pulmonary venous return to left atrium to right ventricle to aorta. Long-term problems with conduction abnormalities and systemic right ventricular failure
Damus–Kaye–Stansel procedure	Main PA is directly anastomosed to the aorta. The branch PAs are supplied by a conduit or a shunt. Augments aortic or sub-aortic hypoplasia/stenosis and provides adequate systemic outflow. Usually in univentricular repair but can be in biventricular repair if RV–PA conduit (Fig. 19.2)
Discordance	A term used in the sequential segmental description of cardiac morphology. Atrioventricular (AV) discordance, e.g. right atrium connects to the left ventricle (NB the AV valve relates to the ventricle therefore this would be a mitral valve). Ventriculo-arterial discordance, e.g. left ventricle connects to the PA
Double inlet ventricle	>50% of each AV valve connects to one ventricle (usually left ventricle)

(Continued)

Table 19.1 (Continued)

Term	Description
Double outlet ventricle	>50% of each great vessel arises from one ventricle (usually right ventricle)
Eisenmenger syndrome	Congenital heart defect that initially causes a major left-to-right shunt, induces severe pulmonary vascular disease and pulmonary arterial hypertension, and then finally causes reversal of the shunt with consequent cyanosis
Fenestration	Iatrogenic connection in interatrial, interventricular, or baffled septum allowing right-to-left shunt in context of raised pulmonary vascular resistance, improving cardiac output but at the expense of cyanosis
Fontan procedure (Fig. 19.7)	Systemic venous return is connected to the pulmonary arteries without ventricular pump. Original operation described connection of the right atrial appendage to the PA. Contemporary operations have extracardiac and intracardiac (e.g. lateral tunnel) conduit variations. Most have a small fenestration that allows for a small right-to-left shunt
Glenn connection	Superior vena cava (SVC) connected to PA. Bidirectional Glenn describes the SVC connecting to confluent (connected) right and left pulmonary arteries
Hemitruncus	Right or left branch PA originating from the aorta
Konno procedure	Operation to enlarge aortic annulus and left ventricular outflow tract (LVOT). LVOT enlarged with patch through right ventriculotomy. Complications include heart block and ventricular septal defect
Left SVC	Persistence of connection from left subclavian vein and coronary sinus. Coronary sinus usually dilated. If coronary sinus unroofed or fenestrated may act as potential source of right-to-left shunt
Mustard procedure (Fig. 19.5)	Atrial switch procedure for transposition of the great arteries. The atrial septum is resected and then an intra-atrial baffle of pericardial tissue constructed to divert systemic venous return to the mitral annulus and then the sub-pulmonary left ventricle. Long-term complications include atrial arrhythmias and systemic right ventricular failure
Norwood procedure	Palliative series of operations for hypoplastic left heart syndromes achieving a single ventricle repair with systemic RV Stage I: highly complex procedure that achieves connection of PA to aorta to enlarge outflow, shunt from aorta to PAs, and atrial septectomy Stage II: shunt taken down and bidirectional Glenn procedure Stage III: completion of Fontan procedure
Pott shunt	Palliative shunt connecting the descending aorta to the left PA

(Continued)

Table 19.1 (Continued)

Term	Description
Rastelli operation	Specific procedure for transposition of the great arteries, with ventricular septal defect and pulmonary stenosis. Left ventricular outflow is baffled through a ventricular septal defect to the malpositioned aorta. A tube graft connects the right ventricle to the PA
Ross procedure	Replacement of aortic valve with native pulmonary valve (autograft). A homograft replaces the pulmonary valve. Utilized particularly in children to facilitate graft growth. Long-term potential problems with autograft and homograft failure. May require LVOT enlargement, i.e. Ross–Konno procedure
Senning procedure	Intra-atrial baffling of venous return in transposition of the great arteries. Similar to the Mustard procedure but using atrial tissue and no prosthetic material
Single ventricle	Also known as univentricular. Functionally one pumping chamber, although there is often a vestigial remnant of a second ventricular chamber
Straddling	Valve with chordal attachments crossing a ventricular septal defect, thus limiting definitive repair
Subclavian aortoplasty	Surgical repair of coarctation of the aorta using the left subclavian artery to patch augment the coarctation segment. Resultant reduction or absence of palpable pulses or measureable BP in the left arm
Switch operation (Fig. 19.6)	Surgical repair for transposition of the great arteries restoring ventriculo-arterial concordance by an arterial switch repair of the great vessels with transfer of coronary arteries to the aorta. Long-term issues include stenoses at pulmonary, aortic, or coronary anastomoses or branch PA stenoses
Tetralogy of Fallot (Fig. 19.1)	Key features are ventricular septal deviation with aortic override and right ventricular outflow tract obstruction with consequent right ventricular hypertrophy. Primary repair now more common, but if unstable and cyanotic maybe palliated with shunts (Blalock–Taussig, Waterston or Pott) to allow growth. Long-term issues include pulmonary valve regurgitation or stenosis, right ventricular dilatation, and ventricular tachyarrhythmias
Total cavopulmonary connection (Fig. 19.8)	Also known as a TCPC. Contemporary variation of the Fontan procedure with SVC connected to PA (Glenn connection) and IVC connected to the PA usually via an extra-cardiac connection
Transposition of the great arteries (Fig. 19.4)	Ventriculo-arterial discordance: aorta arises from right ventricle
Truncus arteriosus	Single vessel outlet from the heart from which aortic and pulmonary arterial flows then develop
Waterston shunt	Palliative shunt connecting the ascending aorta and right PA

Reproduced from Matthew Barnard and Bruce Martin, *Oxford Specialist Handbook: Cardiac Anaesthesia*, 2010, Table 30.1, with permission from Oxford University Press.

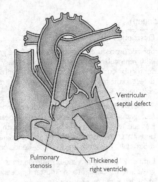

Figure 19.1 Tetralogy of Fallot. Reproduced with kind permission from Yorkshire and Humber Adult Congenital Heart Disease Network.

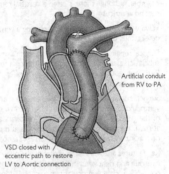

Figure 19.2 RV–PA conduit. Reproduced with kind permission from Yorkshire and Humber Adult Congenital Heart Disease Network.

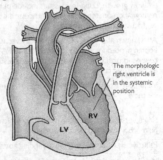

Figure 19.3 Congenitally corrected transposition of the great arteries (CCTGA). Reproduced with kind permission from Yorkshire and Humber Adult Congenital Heart Disease Network.

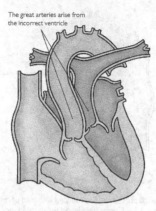

The great arteries arise from the incorrect ventricle

Figure 19.4 Transposition of the great arteries (TGA). Reproduced with kind permission from Yorkshire and Humber Adult Congenital Heart Disease Network.

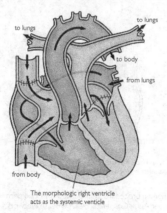

to lungs

to lungs

to body

from lungs

from body

The morphologic right ventricle acts as the systemic venticle

Figure 19.5 The Mustard repair. Reproduced with kind permission from Yorkshire and Humber Adult Congenital Heart Disease Network.

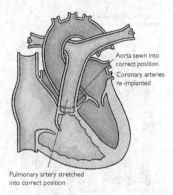

Aorta sewn into
correct position

Coronary arteries
re-implanted

Pulmonary artery stretched
into correct position

Figure 19.6 The Switch procedure. Reproduced with kind permission from
Yorkshire and Humber Adult Congenital Heart Disease Network.

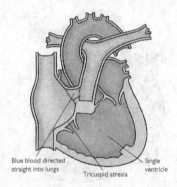

Blue blood directed
straight into lungs

Tricuspid atresia

Single
ventricle

Figure 19.7 The Fontan procedure. Reproduced with kind permission from
Yorkshire and Humber Adult Congenital Heart Disease Network.

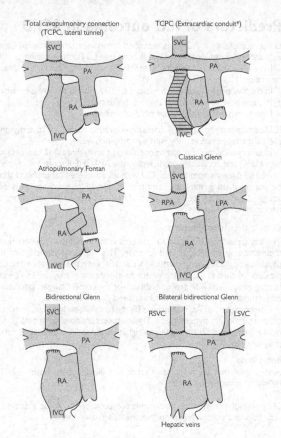

Figure 19.8 Total cavopulmonary connection (TCPC). Reproduced from SG Myerson et al., *Emergencies in Cardiology*, 2006, p. 243, with permission from Oxford University Press.

Predictors of ICU outcome in ACHD

Lesion complexity in ACHD is described according to the Canadian Cardiovascular Society's Consensus Classification (see 📖 Further reading, p. 198).

Increasing lesion complexity is associated with higher ICU morbidity and mortality:

In elective postoperative admissions to ICU morbidity increases with:
- Preoperative renal, liver, or thyroid dysfunction
- Haemodynamically significant residual lesions.

ICU admissions prompted by acute deterioration secondary to arrhythmias can be managed successfully with a good outcome.

In emergency medical admissions (except arrhythmias) ICU mortality is high (36%) and accurately predicted by the APACHE II score.

ACHD patients admitted to ICU with an acute medical problem should be managed using standard principles of care. However, advice is often sought from CICU specialists particularly with regard to ventilatory and haemodynamic support.

General considerations

The key factor to CICU care for patients with ACHD is an appreciation of their anatomy, physiology, and function. This includes knowledge of their usual haemoglobin, oxygen saturation, and BP. Even this can reveal the complexities of care as identifying where to measure the 'true' BP can be challenging in a patient with previous shunts, or the correct oxygen saturation in an Eisenmenger patient with an unrepaired ductus arteriosus.

Complications of ACHD include RV dysfunction, arrhythmia, endocarditis, and pulmonary hypertension. These aspects are covered in detail in their relevant chapters. Chapter 20 also highlights the specific aspects of care of pregnancy in ACHD.

Arrhythmias

Arrhythmias may be difficult to detect. Knowledge of the baseline ECG is helpful.

> Any arrhythmia with haemodynamic compromise should be managed in the standard way, with prompt electrical cardioversion.

Atrial tachyarrhythmias are life-threatening to patients with single ventricular physiologies. If an atrial tachyarrhythmia is diagnosed then prompt action is required to manage the patient:
- *Electrical cardioversion* is treatment of choice.
- Amiodarone can potentially slow the rate of atrial conduction and risk 1:1 AV conduction with consequent haemodynamic collapse.

Cyanosis

Cyanosis is an important feature of unrepaired or some palliated ACHD syndromes. Hypoxaemia is caused by right-to-left shunts or mixing of pulmonary venous and systemic venous returns in a common chamber. A secondary erythrocytosis results with an elevated haematocrit and subsequent hyperviscosity.

- Preoperatively efforts should be made to optimize iron stores to ensure that the patient is iron-replete with optimal haemoglobin for their physiology.
- Venesection is very infrequently performed; essentially only if symptomatic hyperviscosity syndrome.
- Cyanotic patients are at risk of systemic emboli: new neurological findings should prompt urgent brain imaging for potential cerebral emboli.
- Chronic cyanosis has many sequelae including; haemostatic abnormalities, renal impairment, and development of aorto-pulmonary collateral arteries.
- Cyanotic patients often have a coagulopathy associated with thrombocytopenia consequent to their secondary erythrocytosis. There are also some reports of ↓ levels of coagulation factors V, VII, VIII, and IX and reduced von Willebrand multimers.
- The patient may develop critically compromised oxygen delivery perioperatively due to hypovolaemia or relative anaemia. Transfusion may be required, not to a specific target haemoglobin, but rather to achieve adequate oxygen delivery.

Haemoptysis may be life threatening. If Eisenmenger physiology, remember that systemic and pulmonary pressures are similar; if hypertensive, avoid vasodilators, and treat with β-blockers ± sedation.

Haemoptysis

Haemoptysis is a worrying symptom in ACHD. A small-volume bleed may be the herald of a life-threatening haemoptysis and so should be investigated thoroughly. The source of bleed may be related to bronchitis, PE, and in pulmonary hypertensive patients, pulmonary arterial rupture or rupture of an aorto-pulmonary collateral vessel. In patients with tracheostomy or prolonged ventilation a tracheo-arterial fistula may form. In patients with aortic aneurysm including coarctation repairs and Marfan syndrome there may be erosion into the airway (or oesophagus).

Prompt investigation includes CXR, bronchoscopy, CT angiography, and invasive catheterization with the potential of embolizing the bleeding vessel.
   If major bleeding, consider selective intubation of non-bleeding bronchus or bronchial blocker.

Heart failure

Patients with ACHD may develop heart failure. This should be managed according to standard management strategies although there is less evidence of benefit, particularly in systemic right ventricles.
   The evidence for cardiac resynchronization therapy (CRT) in ACHD is minimal but it can be considered in specific cases, and may be appropriate in the CICU setting where a patient may have become pacing dependent postoperatively and subsequently develops systemic ventricular failure. Access to achieve CRT may be challenging and may require an epicardial lead to be positioned.

Advanced heart failure strategies may be required, including mechanical circulatory support and transplantation. In the postoperative period ACHD patients may require ECMO support or a VAD. VAD technology has been a significant advance in the postoperative management of right ventricular dysfunction in the ACHD population. Cardiac transplantation in ACHD patients is appropriate for consideration, but requires significant technical consideration and planning.

General principles in care of patients with ACHD

- The aim of care is to achieve adequate end-organ oxygen delivery.
- Oxygen therapy is not harmful to patients with ACHD. Therefore oxygen can be used as in general patients. However, oxygen saturations should be monitored with consideration of the patient's usual saturation.
- Meticulous care of IV access should be maintained to avoid bubbles. Air bubbles may enter the systemic circulation. Similarly, cerebral abscesses may form due to paradoxical emboli into the systemic circulation. New neurological signs should be investigated with advanced brain imaging.
- Invasive monitoring requires consideration. Arterial access should be sited to avoid pressure damping from previous shunts or coarctation repairs. Central venous lines should avoid cavopulmonary connections as these connect directly with the pulmonary arteries. Pulmonary artery flotation catheters are fraught with problems in the ACHD patient and often cause more problems than they solve: in general they should be avoided.

Further reading

Price S, Jaggar SI, Jordan S, Trenfield S, Khan M, Sethia B, *et al*. Adult congenital heart disease: intensive care management and outcome prediction. *Intensive Care Med* 2007;33:652–9.
Warnes CA, Liberthson R, Danielson GK, Dore A, Harris L, Hoffman JI, et al. Task force 1: the changing profile of congenital heart disease in adult life. *JACC*. 2001;37:1170–5.

Lesion-specific considerations

Tetralogy of Fallot

The most common cause of planned ICU admission in adults with Tetralogy of Fallot is re-do surgery for pulmonary valve replacement. In planning these patients monitoring in ICU attention should be paid to previous surgeries:

- If a patient has had previous Blalock–Taussig shunts then they are likely to have a falsely low arterial BP in the arm on the same side as the thoracotomy scar.
- Many patients will recover promptly from their surgery, however there is potential for ICU complications.
- *RV dysfunction* frequently causes morbidity and this should be promptly managed using the strategies described in 📖 Management of the failing RV, pp. 88: optimization of ventilation, ensure heart rate and rhythm are optimal, preload optimization, modification of afterload including early use of nitric oxide, and consideration of advanced mechanical support.
- The role of inter-ventricular dependence in *LV dysfunction* is unclear, but additional factors in LV dysfunction include coronary artery disease. LV dysfunction should be managed with standard heart failure strategies.
- *Arrhythmias* are potentially problematic and need prompt attention. Sustained ventricular arrhythmias may require electrical cardioversion. Optimization of electrolytes and consideration of anti-arrhythmic agents including amiodarone may be required in the acute setting, and a proportion of the tetralogy patients require implantable defibrillators pre-discharge.

Transposition of the great arteries—Mustard or Senning repair

Surgery in adults with previous Mustard or Senning repair may be for obstructed or leaking baffles. They are likely to have postoperative renal and hepatic dysfunction secondary to chronic venous congestion that may be slow to resolve.

- *Systemic RV dysfunction* is often challenging to manage. Standard heart failure strategies should be instigated although the response is not predictable.

Transposition of the great arteries—switch repair

Operative indications in patients with previous arterial switch include repair of the pulmonary, aortic, or coronary artery anastomoses, or valve repair or replacement of the aortic or pulmonary valves.

- The major concern in these patients is systemic left ventricular failure often due to coronary ischaemia.

Congenitally corrected transposition of the great arteries

There are two frequent presentations of adults with CCTGA: bradyarrhythmia requiring pacemaker, and systemic atrioventricular (tricuspid) valve regurgitation. Tricuspid valve regurgitation may be a manifestation of systemic RV failure, and this may be challenging to manage in the postoperative period. These patients may require support from a VAD.

Fontan and TCPC circulations

The Fontan circulation is a univentricular physiology which depends on passive pulmonary blood flow. IPPV will drop the cardiac output compared with spontaneous breathing, by preventing the negative intrathoracic pressure generated during inspiration which increases pulmonary blood flow. Cardiac output in the Fontan physiology requires an adequate preload and avoidance of elevated pulmonary vascular resistance.

• Avoidance of IPPV is preferred, however IPPV can be tolerated if the change in cardiac output is anticipated and managed. The lowest airway pressures should be utilized with minimal PEEP. Early extubation is advocated but not at the risk of airway compromise.

• Fontan physiology is associated with systemic venous hypertension with chronic changes in renal, liver, and haematological function all of which are challenging in the postoperative setting.

In the CICU setting Fontan patients require careful management. In addition to the systemic problems already described, potential cardiovascular problems include:

• *Systemic ventricular dysfunction*: manage with standard strategies. Preliminary evidence suggests that calcium sensitizers such as levosimendan may be beneficial. Maximizing cardiac output may require aggressive management of pleural effusions and ascites (which may splint diaphragmatic function), optimization of ventilator parameters in combination with bronchodilatation and reduction of pulmonary vascular resistance with pulmonary vasodilators (potentially in combination for maximal effect).

• *Arrhythmias*: Fontan heart rate is usually between 40–90bpm. Atrial arrhythmias may be difficult to discern from usual rhythm. Atrial ECG may be possible postoperatively. Arrhythmias are poorly tolerated and prompt electrical cardioversion should be considered.

Conclusion

• The management of ACHD patients in CICU is complex and challenging, but highly rewarding in terms of the impact on a young population.

• Information about the past history and contemporary investigations is key to appreciating the current anatomy and physiology.

• Support and advice should be sought from ACHD specialists—cardiologists, cardiac surgeons, anaesthetists, and intensivists.

Further reading

Griffiths M, Cordingley J, Price S (eds). *Cardiovascular Critical Care*. Oxford: Wiley-Blackwell; 2010.

The obstetric patient with cardiac disease

Introduction

Cardiac disease can complicate pregnancy and can result in admission to a critical care unit. The most recent CMACE report 2006–2008 reported 2.3 deaths per 100,000 maternities (Fig. 20.1). Cardiac causes remain first in the list of causes of maternal death (Fig. 20.2). Increasingly women with severe cardiac disease are opting for pregnancy with the expectation of good maternal and neonatal outcomes. This presents huge challenges for obstetric services and good outcomes are dependent on cardiac obstetric networks including excellent cardiac critical care.

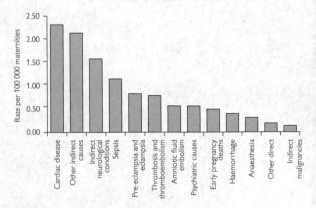

Figure 20.1 Leading causes of maternal death per 100,000 maternities, UK: 2006–2008. Other indirect causes are separated into neurological and other, and other direct included fatty liver and direct cancer. Reproduced from Lewis, G. et al., *Saving mothers' lives: reviewing maternal deaths to make motherhood safer: 2006–2008, BJOG: An International Journal of Obstetrics and Gynaecology*, 118, s1, pp. 1–203, Wiley, © 2011 Centre for Maternal and Child Enquiries (CMACE), BJOG.

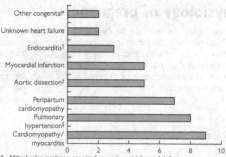

* Miltral valve prolapse, repaired secundum atrial septal defect
† Repaired coarctation, bicuspid aortic valve, normal heart
‡ 2 Marfan, 2 previously normal, 1 hypertension
§ 3 Primary, 2 Eisenmenger, 1 repaired atrial septal defect and pulmonary hypertension, 1 talc granuloma, 1 unknown

Figure 20.2 Cardiac causes of maternal deaths in the UK: confidential enquiry into maternal deaths 1997–1999 (total maternal deaths = 409, cardiac deaths = 41). Reproduced from *Heart and Education in Heart*, SA Thorne, Pregnancy in heart disease, 90, 4, pp. 450–456, copyright 2004, with permission from BMJ Publishing Group Ltd.

The physiology of pregnancy

Pregnancy makes great demands on the cardiac function during pregnancy (Fig. 20.3). Patients with limited cardiac reserve can decompensate during pregnancy risking both maternal and fetal well-being. Complications can occur for up to several days after delivery. In the immediate aftermath of delivery there is an autotransfusion of placental blood which may precipitate cardiac volume overload.

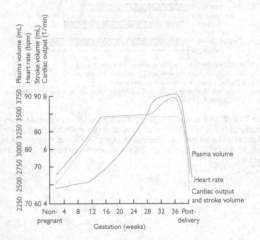

Figure 20.3 Physiological changes in pregnancy. Systemic and pulmonary vascular resistance (PVR) fall during pregnancy. BP may fall in the 2nd trimester, rising slightly in late pregnancy. Note that cardiac output and stroke volume peak by 16 weeks of gestation. Reproduced from *Heart and Education in Heart*, SA Thorne, Pregnancy in heart disease, 90, 4, pp. 450–456, copyright 2004, with permission from BMJ Publishing Group Ltd.

The risk of maternal death

Antenatal advice should be given to patients with significant cardiac disease. Exact prediction of maternal and fetal outcomes can be difficult with the progressive advances in medical care and the limited experience of pregnancy in rare cardiac diseases.

Mothers with complex cardiac disease should attend a joint clinic with a specialist cardiologist and the high-risk pregnancy obstetric team. The role of the clinic is to assess and advise the mother on the risk of pregnancy and to develop a plan to minimize these risks through close follow-up and medical intervention.

Patients at high risk of cardiac mortality should be delivered in a hospital which can provide specialist cardiac obstetric services (Table 20.1). After delivery, close supervision and treatment in a cardiac critical care unit is beneficial.

Table 20.1 Risk of maternal death in ACHD

Condition	Risk of death
Normal healthy woman	1 in 20,000
Average for the population	1 in 10,000
Corrected Fallot's or similar	1 in 1000
Severe aortic stenosis	1 in 100
Severe pulmonary hypertension	1 in 3
Eisenmenger's complex	1 in 2

Reproduced from MA Gatzoulis et al., *Adult congenital heart disease: A practical guide*, Copyright ©
2005 by Blackwell Publishing Ltd, with permission.

Independent predictors of cardiac risk are:
- Cyanotic heart disease
- Pulmonary hypertension
- Poor functional status (New York Heart Association (NYHA) III or IV)
- Poor systemic ventricular function
- Severe left sided obstruction.

More patients with congenital heart disease are surviving to adulthood and
are wishing to risk pregnancy. Eisenmenger's syndrome is known to carry a
major risk with published maternal mortality rates of 40–50%. These types
of patients require preoperative counselling of the risks involved. Complex
cardiac disease in pregnancy is a classic example of a clinical condition
where careful planning and excellent teamwork between multiple disciplines is required. These include obstetricians, cardiologists, paediatricians,
midwifes, anaesthetists, and intensivists. Obstetric patients with complex
cardiac disease should be managed in specialist units with an experienced
cardiac obstetric team and access to cardiac critical care facility.

Medical interventions are sometimes indicated to improve maternal
and neonatal outcome during pregnancy, such as mitral balloon valvuloplasty, coarctation repair, and treatment with anticoagulants or pulmonary
vasodilators.

Anaesthetic techniques and the delivery

The gestation and method of delivery will be determined by the high-risk obstetric team depending on fetal growth and well-being and the cardiac assessment of the mother. In complex cardiac disease, the mother and fetus are assessed serially. The cardiac demands increase as pregnancy progresses; however, this has to be balanced against the fetal risk of premature delivery and the growth and maturity of the baby.

In moderate-risk pregnancies a spontaneous delivery is preferred; however, in high-risk patients a caesarean section may be the delivery method of choice.

The anaesthetic technique will be decided by the responsible anaesthetist depending on a host of factors. Awake regional anaesthesia is the preferred option adopted by many centres.

Basic principles

- Lateral tilt at all times to minimize caval compression from gravid uterus.
- Careful administration of Syntocinon® (5 units IV slowly) post delivery.
- Very cautious fluid administration.
- Vasopressor infusion for spinal anaesthesia. Phenylephrine is our preference.
- Full cardiac backup should be available for the high-risk cardiac obstetric caesarean section. This should include the option of cardiac surgical intervention and/or mechanical support.

Benefits of regional technique

- Mother is awake
- Lower risk of aspiration
- Avoid general anaesthetic side effects
- Good pain relief.

Commonly accepted exceptions to the use of regional technique

- Severe left-sided obstruction (aortic or mitral stenosis)
- Severe cardiomyopathy
- Spinal/combined spinal epidural contraindicated by an absolute contraindication such as dual antiplatelet therapy or anticoagulation.

Benefits of general anaesthesia

- Avoid side effects of regional anaesthesia, i.e. vasodilation
- Control of ventilation
- Easier to escalate support and insert lines.
- TOE monitoring possible.

Risks of general anaesthesia

- CVS depression and decompensation
- Raised intrathoracic pressure
- ↑ PVR
- ↑ uterine atony
- Neonatal depression
- Pulmonary aspiration.

Special consideration for cardiac intensive care

Careful planning of postoperative care is essential. While specialist cardiac intensive care may be lifesaving, all the facilities of an obstetric unit should be available in the peripartum period. This plan should include consideration of the following:

- Appropriate level of CVS monitoring:
  - Arterial pressure
  - Central venous pressure
  - Urinary output
  - Cardiac output
  - SvO_2
  - PA pressures
  - Echo if required
- Analgesia:
  - Paracetamol
  - NSAIDs
  - Epidural or spinal opiates
  - Rescue oral opiate analgesia
- Bleeding complications:
  - Reduced uterine tone treated with routine Syntocinon® infusion
  - Ergometrine
  - Carboprost for uncontrolled postpartum haemorrhage (PPH)
  - The availability of obstetric surgical team
  - Interventional radiology capacity for uncontrollable PPH
  - Hysterectomy may be required if all else fails.
- Antibiotic prophylaxis according to local protocol
- VTE prophylaxis should be given
- Emotional support:
  - Separation from newborn baby is difficult for mother
  - Webcam can help view baby in neonatal ICU
  - Moral support throughout from partner
- Cardiac arrest in the pregnant patient:
  - Resuscitation should follow ERC guidelines
  - Emergency caesarean section within 5 minutes of cardiac arrest
  - Lateral tilt
  - Cricoid pressure for intubation as ↑ risk of aspiration.

Heart failure resistant to standard medical therapy

Introduction

Decompensated heart failure (DHF) is common. The majority of patients with DHF respond well to standard medical therapy, however some do not, experiencing worsening signs and symptoms. This chapter will focus on the assessment and general management of patients where standard medical therapy is failing and more advanced options are required. These are intravenous inotropic therapy, intra-aortic balloon pump (IABP) counter-pulsation, ultrafiltration, formal mechanical circulatory support (MCS), and/or cardiac transplantation. Further information on these specific strategies will be found in respective individual chapters.

Presentation

Heart failure may be new or an exacerbation of chronic disease. The clinical syndrome is characterized by breathlessness associated with accumulation of fluid within the lung's interstitial and alveolar spaces resulting from elevated cardiac filling pressures. Other organ dysfunction may be present and the patient may be hypotensive (cardiogenic shock). HF is most commonly due to LV systolic or diastolic dysfunction; other cardiac abnormalities may also exist such as coronary artery or valvular disease.

Specialist versus non-specialist care

The recognition and management of patients refractory to standard medical care is challenging and ideally such patients are best managed in specialized CICUs which can provide a full range of options. However, most patients will present to more generalist units and be managed outside intensive care. The identification of the at-risk subgroup, the decision to refer, and the timing of transfer are crucial. Early consultation with specialist units should be encouraged, if possible as part of a formal clinical network and underpinned by formal protocols and good clinical relationships.

Assessment

Factors which may precipitate decompensation
- Patient compliance
- Acute medical condition, e.g. lower respiratory tract infection
- Delay in diagnosing DHF
- Arrhythmia, for example, AF or ventricular tachycardia
- Fluid resuscitation at point of admission
- Use of a β-blocker.

History
Can be challenging in presence of of respiratory distress or depressed conscious level. Use accompanying relative or carer if necessary.
Priorities:
- Clarify diagnosis:
  - Is this heart failure or a mimic? (see Table 21.1)
  - Has heart failure been diagnosed previously?
  - Is there dual pathology? e.g. heart failure and pneumonia

Table 21.1 Differential diagnosis of cardiac failure

Respiratory	COPD
	Asthma
	Pulmonary thromboembolism (acute or chronic)
	ARDS
	Pneumonia
	Pulmonary haemorrhage
	Interstitial (fibrotic) lung disease
	Re-expansion pulmonary oedema (pneumothorax)
	Pulmonary veno-occlusive disease
Renal dysfunction	Acute or chronic kidney disease
	Nephrotic syndrome
	Bilateral renal artery stenosis
Drugs (fluid retention/ oedema)	NSAIDS
	Dihydropyridine calcium channel antagonists
'High output cardiac failure'	Severe anaemia
	Thyrotoxicosis
	Thiamine deficiency (beriberi)
	Sepsis
	Arterio-venous shunting
	Paget's disease
Hepatic dysfunction	
Hypoalbuminaemia	
Chronic venous insufficiency	
Neurogenic pulmonary oedema	Intracerebral haemorrhage
	Electroconvulsive therapy
	Head injury
Drug overdose	Opiate toxicity
	Salicylate toxicity

- Assess symptoms:
  - Breathlessness, orthopnoea, paroxysmal nocturnal dyspnoea
  - Grade effort tolerance using the New York Heart Association (NYHA) classification

  - Peripheral oedema: often not present, especially in younger patients despite considerable relative fluid overload due to undetected ascites and bowel oedema

  - Abdominal swelling (ascites), tightness, and bloating
  - Weight changes:
    - —Gain: fluid retention
    - —Loss: cardiac cachexia

- Try to define cause for decompensation or acute presentation:
  - Symptoms of ischaemia, arrhythmia, hypotension
  - Recent medication changes or compliance issues
  - Cardiotoxic drugs or drugs that may exacerbate fluid retention (see Box 21.1)
  - Non-adherence to fluid, salt, or alcohol restriction
  - Beware of the 'nil by mouth' surgical patient. Has cardiac medication been withheld? Has patient received excessive IV fluid?
- Define comorbidities:
  - Associated with worse prognosis (see Box 21.2).
  - Can impact on transplant candidacy (see Chapter 22)
- Establish usual quality of life and whether an advanced directive is in place. Wishes of patient should be of central importance.

Box 21.1 **Potentially reversible cardiac depressants**
- Acidosis
- Sepsis
- Hypoxia
- Drugs with negative inotropic effects: e.g. calcium channel antagonists, most anti-arrhythmic agents, overdose.

Box 21.2 **Common non-cardiac comorbidities in patients with heart failure**
- Anaemia
- Renal dysfunction
- Diabetes mellitus
- COPD
- Arthritis
- Cognitive dysfunction
- Depression.

Examination
Airway, breathing, circulation, disability, exposure (ABCDE).

General
- Does the patient look unwell?
- Skeletal muscle loss may indicate cardiac cachexia.

Cardiovascular
- Pulse and peripheries:
  - Low volume with cool, cyanosed peripheries (peripheral vasoconstriction)
  - Capillary refill
  - Tachycardia: found in most patients with DHF often despite rate limiting medication
  - AF: cause or consequence of decompensation

- BP:
  - Usually low but may be normal or high, especially if hypertension is the underlying cause of heart failure
  - Pulsus paradoxus may indicate cardiac tamponade
- Jugular venous pressure (JVP):
  - Elevated JVP reflecting high cardiac filling pressures
  - Beware of other causes of elevated JVP: tricuspid regurgitation, PE, cardiac tamponade, constrictive pericarditis, right ventricular infarction, obstruction of the SVC
- Praecordium:
  - Palpation: diffuse, laterally displaced apex beat (LV dilatation); RV heave (elevated pulmonary artery pressures or right heart failure)
- Auscultation:
  - 3rd heart sound ('gallop rhythm')
  - Pansystolic murmur of mitral regurgitation
  - The presence of any murmur may indicate valvular pathology, or a septal defect, in the aetiology.

Respiratory
- Tachypnoea at rest
- Bibasal crepitations although absence does not exclude pulmonary oedema
- Pleural effusions.

Abdominal
- Tender hepatomegaly caused by liver congestion and right heart failure is common.

Oedema
- A cardinal feature of cardiac failure but has many other causes and does not correlate well with systemic venous pressure. Often absent in acute *de novo* heart failure and in young heart failure patients.

Investigation
Clinical haematology and biochemistry
- Full blood count: anaemia can exacerbate cardiac failure and, occasionally, is the primary cause of it.
- Renal dysfunction is common and often improves (paradoxically) with aggressive diuretic therapy.
- Electrolytes: frequently disturbed either as a consequence of the disease or, more commonly, as a result of treatment.
- Glucose, lipids, and thyroid function.
- Liver function tests: often abnormal as a result of hepatic congestion caused by cardiac failure.
- Clotting screen: hepatic congestion in heart failure often associated with deranged coagulation parameters.
- Cardiomyopathy 'screen': should be checked when the underlying diagnosis has not been ascertained. Should include:
  - Viral serology (viral myocarditis/cardiomyopathy), ferritin (haemochromatosis), thyroid function tests, calcium, serum ACE (cardiac sarcoidosis), 24-hour urine collection for metanephrines

(phaeochromocytoma), creatine kinase (neuromuscular disease), auto-antibodies (connective tissue disease).
* Troponin: may be marked elevated in myocardial ischaemia and infarction. However, modest elevations also occur in DHF (whatever the cause), myocarditis, and severe non-cardiac illness, e.g. pneumonia.
* Natriuretic peptides such as brain natriuretic peptide (BNP) and its precursor N-terminal-pro BNP (NT-proBNP). Released in response to myocardial wall stress. May help guide therapy in DHF. BNP should fall as condition improves.

Electrocardiogram

* Rarely normal in heart failure. Normal ECG carries a negative predictive value of ~98%.

* Can provide important clues to the underlying aetiology of the cardiac failure:
  * Pathological Q waves and ST segment or T wave changes: suggest the presence of ischaemic heart disease.
  * Large voltage QRS complexes suggest LV hypertrophy.
  * Low voltage QRS complexes: consider hypothyroidism, amyloidosis or pericardial effusion.
  * Electrical alternans: alternating amplitude of QRS complex sometimes seen with pericardial effusion.
* Provides evidence of conduction problems or arrhythmia:
  * Bradycardia or 2nd- or 3rd-degree AV block: cause may be organic conduction system disease or drug side effects.
  * Atrial arrhythmias: particularly common and may either be a cause or a consequence of heart failure.

Chest X-ray
* CXR can often confirm or refute the diagnosis, may provide clues to aetiology, provide alternative diagnoses or highlight complications or comorbidity such as superimposed pneumonia (see Table 21.2).
* Beware: normal cardiothoracic ratio has low sensitivity and specificity for the detection of heart failure (normal in ~40–50% of patients with LV dysfunction).
* Be careful: the relationship between haemodynamic and pulmonary vascular abnormalities are variable. Some patients with severe heart failure may not have X-ray features of pulmonary venous congestion or oedema despite very high pulmonary capillary pressures.

Echocardiography (transthoracic and/or transoesophageal)
* The echocardiogram remains one of the most important investigations in the patient with heart failure. It can detect the presence, the aetiology, and the severity of heart failure. See Chapter 32.

Right heart catheterization
* The utility and appropriateness of right heart catheterization in patients with heart failure is controversial.
* The ESCAPE randomized controlled trial recruited 433 patients with DHF and examined outcomes in those assigned to invasive monitoring

Table 21.2 The CXR in heart failure

Classic CXR features of cardiac failure	CXR features providing clues to the aetiology
Cardiomegaly (cardiothoracic ratio >0.5 (postero-anterior radiograph))	Prominent hilar vessels (pulmonary hypertension)
Upper lobe venous diversion Peribronchial cuffing	Bulging left heart border with retrosternal 'double density' (left ventricular aneurysm)
'Kerley B lines'	Left atrial enlargement (mitral valve disease)
Fluid in horizontal fissure	Pericardial calcification (constrictive pericarditis)
Bilateral alveolar oedema incl. 'bat's wing' perihilar shadowing	Valvular calcification (valvular heart disease)
Pleural effusion (bilateral or R>L)	Rib notching (coarctation of the aorta)

Adapted from Lang NN, Newby DE. Assessment of Patients with Suspected Chronic Heart Failure. In: *Oxford Medical Library: Chronic Heart Failure*. Oxford University Press, UK. 2008.

in the form of right heart catheterization versus those managed by clinical assessment alone. After a 6-month follow-up period there was no difference in the number of days patients were alive and out of hospital and no difference in overall mortality.

- There is no similar data for patients with DHF who require intensive care; many specialist heart failure units consider right heart catheterization an important investigation in this patient group. For example, a normal or low pulmonary artery capillary wedge pressure should question the diagnosis of heart failure and/or may significantly change a frequent model of treatment, aggressive diuresis. Thus, selected patients with severe DHF may benefit from right heart catheterization.
- Right heart catheterization is a routine means of assessment of patients potentially suitable for cardiac transplantation.

Endomyocardial biopsy

- An AHA/ACC/ESC consensus document providing guidance on the appropriateness of endomyocardial biopsy has been published (see Table 21.3). Those scenarios in which biopsy is considered to have a Class I indication primarily focus on the detection or differentiation of giant cell myocarditis from other myocardites for which the prognosis and therapeutic strategy may differ substantially.
- Endomyocardial biopsy might also be considered in heart failure with suspected infiltrative processes such as amyloid, sarcoid, and haemochromatosis, as well as in eosinophilic myocarditis and restrictive cardiomyopathy of unknown origin.
- Cardiac biopsy should only be carried out by operators and centres with experience in performing the procedure.

Table 21.3 Clinical indications for endomyocardial biopsy

Scenario Number	Clinical Scenario	Class of Recommendation (I, IIa, IIb, III)	Level of Evidence (A,B,C)
1	New-onset heart failure of <2 weeks' duration associated with a normal-sized or dilated left ventricle and hemodynamic compromise	I	B
2	New-onset heart failure of 2 weeks' to 3 months' duration associated w/a dilated left ventricle and new ventricular arrhythmias, second- or third-degree heart block, or failure to respond to usual care within 1 to 2 wks	I	B
3	Heart failure of >3 months' duration associated with a dilated left ventricle and new ventricular arrhythmias, second- or third-degree heart block, or failure to respond to usual care within 1 to 2 weeks	IIa	C
4	Heart failure associated with a DCM of any duration associated with suspected allergic reaction and/or eosinophilia	IIa	C
5	Heart failure associated with suspected anthracycline cardiomyopathy	IIa	C
6	Heart failure associated with unexplained restrictive cardiomyopathy	IIa	C
7	Suspected cardiac tumors	IIa	C
8	Unexplained cardiomyopathy in children	IIa	C
9	New-onset heart failure of 2 weeks' to 3 months' duration associated with a dilated left ventricle, without new ventricular arrhythmias or second- or third-degree heart block, that responds to usual care within 1 to 2 weeks	IIb	B
10	Heart failure of >3 months' duration associated with a dilated left ventricle, w/o new ventricular arrhythmias or second- or third-degree heart block, that responds to usual care within 1 1o 2 weeks	IIb	C

(Continued)

Table 21.3 (Continued)

Scenario Number	Clinical Scenario	Class of Recommendation (I, IIa, IIb, III)	Level of Evidence (A,B,C)
11	Heart failure associated with unexplained HCM	IIb	C
12	Suspected ARVD/C	IIb	C
13	Unexplained ventricular arrhythmias	IIb	C
14	Unexplained atrial fibrillation	III	C

Reproduced from LT Cooper et al., 'The role of endomyocardial biopsy in the management of cardiovascular disease: a scientific statement from the American Heart Association, the American College of Cardiology, and the European Society of Cardiology', Circulation, 116, 19, pp. 2216–2233, copyright 2007, with permission from the American Heart Association.

Initial management

- Airway assessment
- Ensure adequate oxygenation (continuous pulse oximetry). Oxygen supplementation can be titrated in order to keep the patient comfortable and arterial oxygen saturation >90%. This can be provided by:
  - Non-rebreather face mask delivering high-flow defined per cent oxygen.
  - Non-invasive positive pressure ventilation (NIV). If respiratory acidosis, respiratory distress, and/or hypoxia, consider NIV as the preferred initial modality of assisted ventilation as long as the patient does not have a contraindication (see Chapter 26).
  - Conventional mechanical ventilation may be necessary in patients with respiratory failure who do not tolerate or have contraindications to NIV, or in patients who fail NIV (see Chapter 26).
- Repeated assessment of BP.
- Continuous ECG.
- IV access.
- Upright posture.
- Urine output monitoring, preferably with the placement of a urethral catheter.
- Pharmacological VTE prophylaxis (e.g. LMWH) is indicated in patients admitted with decompensated HF who are not already anticoagulated and have no contraindication to anticoagulation.
- Diuretic therapy:
  - Loop diuretics, e.g. furosemide intravenously as a continuous infusion (more controllable than boluses). Start at a dose of 5mg/hour increasing to 10mg/hour and if necessary 20mg/hour until diuresis is achieved.
  - Aim for negative fluid balance between 500mL and 1000mL per 24 hours.
  - Monitor urea and electrolytes closely for hyponatraemia and hypokalaemia. Potassium supplementation may be necessary especially if cardiac rhythm is labile.
- Ultrafiltration:
  - Understandably, there has been some interest in the use of this method in patients with DHF. However, studies are small and although they show improvements in morbidity, such as duration of hospital readmission, no mortality benefits have been shown.
  - The role of ultrafiltration in DHF has yet to be defined and should be used with caution.
- Vasodilator therapy (if BP allows):
  - GTN infusion; start at 5mcg/minute, increase by 5mcg/minute to 20mcg/minute. If no response at 20mcg/minute, may increase by 10–20mcg/minute every 3–5 minutes (generally accepted maximum dose 400mcg/minute).
- Morphine or other mu-opioid.
  - Treats dyspnoea and anxiety and agitation. Avoid over narcotization. 2–5mg as required. Target-controlled remifentanil is good alternative with excellent controllability.

- Avoid or stop:
  - β-blockers (see Box 21.3). If concern regarding tachyarrhythmia consider amiodarone as a substitute.
  - Calcium-channel blockers such as nifedipine, diltiazem, and verapamil have negative inotropic activity and for this reason are generally avoided in patients with heart failure due to systolic dysfunction. Other calcium channel blockers such as felodipine and amlodipine appear to be safe in heart failure and can be used to treat hypertension although this is rarely a problem in patients with heart failure resistant to standard medical therapy.
- Consider CVP monitoring
- Consider right heart catheterization (See 'Right heart catheterization' section in 📖 Introduction, p. 219).

NB Prolonged supine or head-down positioning for central line insertion may precipitate further decompensation or even cardiac arrest

- IV inotropes and vasopressors:
  - Inotropic agents such as dobutamine and/or milrinone may be used in selected patients with severe LV systolic dysfunction and low cardiac output syndrome (reduced peripheral perfusion and end-organ dysfunction) for whom treatment may be restricted by borderline systemic BP or inadequate response to vasodilator and diuretic therapy. Such measures are often temporary and act as a bridge to stabilization and/or more definitive treatment.

Consider intravenous inotropes such as dobutamine or milrinone:
- In DHF patients with severe LV systolic dysfunction with low systemic BP (<90mmHg) despite adequate filling pressures or are unresponsive to or intolerant of IV vasodilators.
- In patients with evidence of fluid overload unresponsive to IV diuretics.

The use of IV inotropes in the context of severe DHF should be accompanied by continuous or frequent BP monitoring and continuous monitoring of cardiac rhythm. If tachyarrhythmias or hypotension occur in response to the use of inotropes, consider withdrawal or dose reduction.

Arrhythmia management
Both supraventricular and ventricular arrhythmias can occur in DHF.

Atrial fibrillation
AF is a common in patients with DHF. The relationship between decompensation and AF include:
- DHF can precipitate AF secondary to ↑ cardiac filling pressures, ↑ left atrial pressure, and subsequent wall stretch.
- In this scenario successful treatment of components of the decompensation such as pulmonary oedema may slow the ventricular rate or precipitate cardioversion to sinus rhythm.
- AF can precipitate decompensation, particularly if the ventricular rate is high.

Box 21.3 β-blockers

β-blockers reduce mortality when used in the long-term management of patients with *stable* heart failure. Thus most patients with known heart failure because of LV systolic dysfunction will be taking a β-blocker prior to hospital admission.

The continuation of β-blockers following admission is reasonable in a patient responding to standard medical therapy. However in unstable patients with DHF, the continuation of β-blockers can result in a poor response to usual medical therapy such as intravenous loop diuretic. Moreover, the initiation of a β-blocker in such an unstable patient can result in cardiogenic shock (negatively inotropic) and is a common cause for the deterioration which results in emergency referral to a tertiary centre for advanced therapies.

Many patients with DHF will have a resting tachycardia in response to the decompensation (as a response to maintain cardiac output in the face of a fixed stroke volume). The temptation to attribute the heart failure to the tachycardia is usually misguided but is often used to justify the use of β-blockers in the decompensated patient.

As a general principle, β-blockers should be avoided in DHF. If rate or rhythm control is necessary for AF or broad complex tachycardia, the use of amiodarone is recommended since it is usually well tolerated in the decompensated patient.

- A rate control strategy is adequate in the first instance using drugs such as amiodarone or digoxin Note: medium- to long-acting β-blockers and non-dihydropyridine calcium channel blockers should be avoided; short-acting formulations of β-blockers such as IV esmolol are sometimes used.
- AF may be chronic and not have a direct association with decompensation.
- Rate control is often the preferred initial strategy for the following reasons:
  - Cardioversion prior to the resolution of acute HF will often be followed by early recurrence of AF because DHF can precipitate AF.
  - AF is often a chronic condition and more often than not poor rate control is a response to decompensation rather than causative.

Heparin should be started prior to cardioversion, if possible.

Ventricular arrhythmias

Ventricular tachycardia in the context of DHF may be life threatening and so prompt electrical cardioversion or defibrillation is often required.

If VT recurs after reversion, antiarrhythmic therapy, particularly with amiodarone may be effective.

Escalation

Intra-aortic balloon pump

IABP represents a reliable and effective device for stabilizing patients with DHF. Nonetheless it is invasive, is not complication free, and renders the patient immobile. Identification of patients who may benefit for IABP can be challenging:

- Patients with cardiogenic pulmonary oedema and cardiogenic shock should be considered candidates for IABP and if necessary formal MCS. They usually have a systolic arterial pressure <90mmHg, a cardiac index <2L/min per m², and a PCWP >18mmHg, despite adequate pharmacological therapy.
- Some patients present so acutely that such invasive measurements are not available and/or their trajectory is towards severe cardiogenic shock and death. Emergency IABP insertion should be considered in such patients.
- IABP may be inserted as a bridge to formal MCS and/or transplantation.
- IABP may be inserted to stabilize DHF, improve renal perfusion, and precipitate a diuresis; following a period of stability they can often be removed safely without the need for reinsertion or further escalation of therapy.

Short-term/long-term VAD

IABPs are frequently effective at stabilizing a patient with cardiogenic shock. However, some will decline despite the presence of an IABP. The use of a short-term VAD or ECMO offers more definitive cardiovascular support and can be used as:

- Bridge to transplantation (BTT).
- Bridge to long-term LVAD implantation if suitable donor organ does not become available whilst BTT.
- Bridge to decision, if neurological status is unknown and might be expected to improve with improved 'cardiac output'. Decision may be to move to BTT or palliation if neurological status poor.
- Bridge to recovery if myocardial recovery is plausible, for example, in myocarditis.
- Bridge to retransplantation in acute allograft rejection post first cardiac transplant.

Femoral vein to femoral artery ECMO

The advantages of ECMO:

- Is that it can provide oxygenation (relevant in a patient with severe pulmonary oedema)
- It leaves the chest untouched making cardiac transplantation and/or long-term LVAD implantation attractive for the future.

Disadvantages include:

- Requirement for powerful anticoagulation increasing bleeding risk
- The period on ECMO is limited to 1–2 weeks
- Finally the cardiac chambers are not decompressed.

An alternative to ECMO is a central short-term VAD. Both left and right hearts can be supported if necessary (BiVAD) for up to 2 months with decompression of the cardiac chambers being possible. Unfortunately central short-term VADs require sternotomy and cardiotomy rendering the patient higher risk for future cardiac surgery if upgrade to a long-term LVAD or transplant is required.

Long-term LVAD

These devices are not usually considered in patients in cardiogenic shock because of the relatively poor outcomes seen in such patients married with the cost of the device in comparison to ECMO or a short-term VAD. Additionally, they only support the left heart and so are dependent on the presence of reasonable RV function.

Transplantation

The most common indication for heart transplantation is severe heart failure refractory to medical therapy. Some patients are ambulatory at home prior to admission for transplantation. However, increasingly transplantation is occurring in patients with decompensated heart failure who are inotrope and/or IABP and/or VAD/ECMO dependent (see 🕮 Heart transplantation, pp. 228–9).

End of life

Recognizing when management should focus on palliation rather than prognosis is important.

Average life expectancy following diagnosis of heart failure is <6 years.

Unpredictability in the course of heart failure makes identifying the end of life in patients with heart failure challenging, whether that be an out-patient or intensive care setting. Identification of patients requiring end of life care and palliation is not easy:

- Seek palliative care team advice (if available) early
- Take into consideration functional status of the patient pre-admission
- Seek advice from cardiologist regarding prognosis:
  - Use multidisciplinary team discussion if available
  - Discuss the issue with the patient
  - Discuss issue with family if patient consents.

Communicating with the patient and family

- The life-limiting nature of heart failure should be acknowledged to patient and family early in care.
- Poor prognosis should be conveyed using a structured and planned 'breaking bad news' conversation. Suggested structure includes:
  - Ask patient what they know
  - Answer any queries they have
  - Convey any pieces of information crucial to decision-making
  - Ask if they have any further questions
  - Confirm that they have understood the key issues
  - Summarize the plan of care from hereon.
- The uncertainty of prognosis estimates should be emphasized.
- Regular daily (and if necessary more frequent) updates to patient and family should be planned.
- Issues that should not be overlooked are cardiopulmonary resuscitation status and the deactivation of implantable cardioverter-defibrillators (discussed in 'Treatment').
- If palliation is feasible outside the ICU, and there is time, consider transfer home, to a hospice, or a favoured ward.
- Remember to offer connection to spiritual services.

Treatment

Key aim is palliation of symptoms.

Thoroughly assess symptoms. Ask whether the patient is experiencing dyspnoea, pain, nausea, sleep disturbance, depression/anxiety, constipation, and anorexia.

Do not wait for patients to volunteer symptoms, consider using a standardized questionnaire.

To avoid repeated shocks, discuss deactivation of implantable cardioverter-defibrillator with patient if relevant. Present turning off the defibrillator function as a simple step to improving the quality of the last few days of life. Emergency deactivation can usually be accomplished by placing a magnet over the defibrillator box; the magnet must remain in place for continued deactivation.

Many standard heart failure treatments are effective at alleviating symptom burden and should be used in palliation/end of life setting. They include:

- Oxygen. Ask the patient what mode of administration they prefer.
- Morphine or other mu-opioid. Treats dyspnoea and anxiety and agitation. Avoid over-narcotization. 2–5 mg as required. Alternatively give as continuous intravenous or subcutaneous infusion.
- Diuretics. Fluid overload should be treated with diuretics such as loop, thiazide, and aldosterone antagonists. Consider oral or intravenous administration. Remember that frusemide can be given subcutaneously if necessary.
- ACE inhibitors, angiotensin II receptor antagonists, and β-blockers. Their role in a dying patient with decompensation is unknown but unlikely to improve symptoms acutely in a patient with end-stage DHF. Indeed, B-blockers are likely to make symptoms worse (see Box 21.3, p. 220). Have a low threshold to withdraw these drugs in palliated patients who are in-patients.

Step down/weaning

- Weaning of inotropes, artificial ventilation, and IABP support is common if a patient's condition improves.
- Commonly, weaning from a ventilator is the first goal, followed by weaning from inotropes, and finally weaning from balloon pump.
- Ventilator weaning (see 📖 Weaning strategies, p. 283).
- Weaning from inotropes (see 📖 Management of hypotension, p. 51).

Weaning from IABP

It is usual practice to lower the frequency of balloon pump inflation prior to removal. For example, 4 hours at one inflation in every two cardiac cycles ('1 in 2') would be the relatively rapid weaning in a patient that might be expected to tolerate removal. Alternatively for patients who have been balloon pump-dependent for several weeks, 24 hours at '1 in 2' then a further 24 hours at '1 in 3' might be a more judicious plan prior to IABP removal. Care should be taken to monitor patients closely in the first 24 hours post IABP removal looking for evidence of decompensation.

The transplant patient

Cardiac transplantation

Cardiac transplantation (CTx) is the final option for patients with heart failure who remain symptomatic despite optimal medical and device therapy. Patients need to be free of significant comorbidities so that they can tolerate major cardiac surgery and subsequent immunosuppression.

Indications for CTx

- Advanced chronic heart failure refractory to maximum tolerated medical, device, or surgical therapy. Patients who benefit have an expected annual mortality rate in excess of 25%.
- Life-threatening acute heart failure unresponsive to initial therapy (e.g. post-MI cardiogenic shock)
- Refractory life-threatening arrhythmias
- Intractable angina not amenable to revascularization or other methods of pain control (uncommon indication).

Prognosis

The 1-year survival following CTx is 85%, with a conditional median survival of 13 years. Patients bridged to CTx with mechanical circulatory support have a higher risk of mortality.

Patient selection for heart transplantation

The selection of patients for CTx is difficult. It is important to identify those at the highest risk of mortality prior to listing, as CTx has a 1-year mortality of ~15%.

Conventional criteria for heart transplantation

- Severe LV systolic function with NYHA class III or IV symptoms
- Optimal medical therapy (maximum doses of β-blockers, ACE inhibitor, aldosterone antagonists) and CRT-P/D or implantable cardioverter defibrillator device implanted (if indicated).
- Evidence of a poor prognosis, e.g.:
  - VO_2 max. <12mL/kg/min (on β-blocker) or <14mL/kg/min (if not on β-blocker), ensuring respiratory exchange ratio ≥1.05
  - Elevated BNP (or NT-proBNP) serum concentration
  - Established composite prognostic scoring system, such as the HFSS or Seattle Heart Failure Model.

Risk factors and contraindications

Whenever possible, intrinsic organ damage should be differentiated from reversible abnormalities secondary to heart failure. Contraindications include:

- Active malignancy (absolute)—collaborate with oncologists
- Active infection (absolute)
- Irreversible pulmonary hypertension (PVR >5 Wood units, transpulmonary gradient >15mmHg)
- Advanced irreversible renal disease (eGFR <40mL/min)
- Advanced irreversible hepatic disease
- Irreversible pulmonary parenchymal disease
- Peripheral or cerebrovascular disease

- Life expectancy markedly compromised by other systemic disease
- Inability to comply with immunosuppressive regimen
- Continuing smoking, alcohol, or substance misuse
- Advanced age (>65 in practice, due to comorbidity)
- Diabetes mellitus with microvascular complications
- Hepatitis B, C, or HIV positive
- Severe obesity (BMI >30)
- Recent PE (i.e. within 3 months)
- Severe osteoporosis.

Immediate post-transplant management

The perioperative management of heart transplant recipients offers several unique challenges to the cardiothoracic intensivist. As well as the usual postoperative problems of bleeding and haemodynamic instability, there is the added burden of:

- Arrhythmia
- Fluid status management
- Bleeding
- Pericardial effusion
- Myocardial stunning due to a long ischaemic time
- RV dysfunction
- Early graft failure
- Immunosuppressive therapy
- Opportunistic infection.

Arrhythmia

Sinus bradycardia and sinus arrest are common. Transient AV block is common but usually resolves within the first few hours.

Management

- Epicardial pacing wires are placed on the atrium and ventricle at the time of surgery. Patients are paced DDD at a rate >110bpm. Daily checks of threshold and sensitivity should be made. See 🕮 Mandatory checks, p. 310.
- Implantation of a permanent pacemaker is required in <5% of recipients.

Fluid status management

- Maintain CVP 5–12mmHg to provide adequate filling without RV overload. Consider colloid replacement in first 24 hours.
- IV loop diuretics by infusion may be required to maintain fluid balance, ± sequential nephronal blockade using thiazide diuretics or aldosterone antagonists.
- CVVH may be required for fluid management.

Bleeding

Of particular concern in patients undergoing redo surgery or following bridging with an LVAD. Early reversal of anticoagulation and the monitoring of haemostatic function with a thromboelastogram can be of assistance in the management of such patients. Platelet transfusion may be required, especially in those who have been receiving dual antiplatelet drug therapy, but the use of blood products may increase PVR and so be associated with a higher risk of right heart failure.

Blood products should be leucocyte depleted. If the donor and recipient are CMV negative, all blood products should also be CMV negative.

Myocardial stunning

The total ischaemic time of the donor heart (cross-clamp on donor heart to cross-clamp off after implantation) is directly correlated with postoperative myocardial performance. While the shorter the time the better, transplant teams aim for an ischaemic time of <4 hours with an ↑ mortality observed for total ischaemic time >5 hours.

Acute RV failure

Frequently seen in the immediate post-bypass period and is of critical importance. RV failure is precipitated by both the transplanted heart being exposed to an ↑ afterload with high PVR and having reduced contractility secondary to myocardial stunning. The RV tends to overdistend, and so loses forward flow down the RCA. Anastomotic complications, such as kinking or torsion at the pulmonary anastomosis, can contribute to postoperative RV dysfunction.

Monitoring

A PAFC should be inserted to allow continuous monitoring of cardiac output and pulmonary artery pressures (PAPs). Some surgeons also use a left atrial line to allow direct monitoring of left-sided filling pressures. TOE is useful in monitoring RV distension.

* High PA pressures with RAP >20mmHg, LAP <10mmHg, and decreasing cardiac output (CO) and mean arterial pressure (MAP).

Management

* Maintain sinus rhythm or pace DDD at a heart rate of over 110bpm. Reducing diastolic time helps to reduce distension of the RV.
* Preload—the RV is very preload sensitive and fluid boluses should be restricted to 50–100mL then re-assessed.
* Inotropic support of RV. Agents are chosen for combined actions:
  * Milrinone is an inotrope which vasodilates the pulmonary vascular bed and reduces systemic vascular tone. Infuse at 0.375–0.75mcg/kg/min.
  * Dobutamine is commonly infused with a low dose of dopamine for their combined inotropy and vasodilatation. Both at 2.5–5mcg/kg/min.
* Reduce afterload. PVR should be managed with inhaled and systemic vasodilator therapy:
  * Inhaled nitric oxide may be used prophylactically in patients known to have ↑ PVR and should be initiated early where there is any sign of right ventricular distension or dysfunction. Start at 20ppm and titrate down.
  * Once it is established the ↑ PVR is reversible, inhaled nitric oxide therapy may be converted to IV or oral therapy. Sildenafil IV 10mg three times daily or oral 20mg three times daily.

Early graft failure

Failure to achieve satisfactory haemodynamics with adequate CO and acceptable filling pressures, without the use of excessive inotropic support, should prompt a complete diagnostic reassessment to exclude technical problems and rejection. Occasionally, short-term support with a VAD (e.g. Levitronix system) or veno-arterial ECMO is necessary to avoid a slide into multisystem organ failure. Retransplantation for acute graft failure early after the original CTx has a 40–60% risk of death at 1 year.

Immunosuppressive therapy

See 📖 Immunosuppression, p. 237.

Opportunistic infection

Prophylactic antibiotics are used in the early postoperative phase.

Cardiac allograft rejection

Rejection can be either cellular or antibody mediated, although in the non-sensitized patient, cellular rejection is the most common form of acute rejection. ISHLT registry data suggests that ~30% of CTx recipients have a rejection episode in the first postoperative year. Risk factors include:
- Female sex
- Younger patients
- Patients receiving immunosuppressive induction therapy.

Patients who do not have an acute rejection episode in the first year have a better 3-year survival (94% vs 88%, p=0.001), and are less likely to develop cardiac allograft vasculopathy.

Early rejection is often asymptomatic but clinical signs suspicious of cardiac allograft rejection include:
- Pyrexia
- Atrial arrhythmias
- Changes in ECG voltage
- 3rd heart sound
- Heart failure.

Endomyocardial biopsy

In 1973, Philip Caves first described transvenous endomyocardial biopsy to diagnose cardiac allograft rejection. Most centres continue to use this technique in the early phase after CTx, when the risk of rejection is highest, and while immunosuppressive therapy is slowly weaned to maintenance doses. This is generally performed from a right internal jugular approach, although the femoral route can be employed with the use of a long venous sheath. An example of a biopsy protocol is:
- Weekly for the first 6 weeks
- Fortnightly from 6 weeks to 3 months
- 6-weekly up to 1 year
- Thereafter only when rejection is clinically suspected.

Potential complications

(Total procedural risk of ~3%.)
- Arrhythmias

- Tamponade
- Tricuspid valve trauma
- Pneumothorax
- Conduction disturbance
- Air embolism
- Nerve palsy.

Treatment of cardiac allograft rejection

(See Table 22.1.)

- Maintain oral immunosuppressive therapy at optimum levels and ensure compliance.
- Grade 1R ACR without evidence of allograft dysfunction does not require further therapy.
- For Grades 2R and 3R ACR, one of the following additional measures is prescribed:
  - Methylprednisolone 1g IV daily for 3 days
  - Antithymocyte globulin (ATG) 0.5mL/kg/day for 3 days
  - Monomurab-CD3 (OKT3).

Table 22.1 The 2005 revision of the Working Formulation for classification of acute cellular rejection of the heart. ACR, acute cellular rejection; R, revised (avoiding confusion with the grades used in the 1990 Working Formulation)

Grade	Category	Description
0	No rejection	–
1R	Mild ACR	Multifocal interstitial and/or perivascular mononuclear infiltrates of lymphocytes, some macrophages and occasional eosinophils ± one focus of myocytolysis
2R	Moderate ACR	Two or more foci of mononuclear cell infiltrates expanding interstitium and with two or more foci of myocyte damage
3R	Severe ACR	Diffuse mononuclear cell infiltrates expanding interstitium ± oedema ± haemorrhage ± neutrophils ± widespread myocyte necrosis ± vasculiti

Reprinted from *The Journal of Heart and Lung Transplantation*, 24, 11, Stewart, S., et al, 'Revision of the 1990 Working Formulation for the Standardization of Nomenclature in the Diagnosis of Heart Rejection', pp.1710–1720, Copyright 2005, with permission from International Society for Heart and Lung Transplantation, and Elsevier.

Lung transplantation

Lung transplantation (LTx) is an option for patients with end-stage lung disease, although the number of available donor organs remains far fewer than the number of patients who would stand to benefit from this procedure. LTx was first performed in 1963 by James Hardy, although the patient only survived for 18 days. Multiple other attempts were thwarted by rejection until Joel Cooper performed the first successful single LTx in 1983, followed by double LTx in 1986.

Indications

Three conditions account for 70% of LTx: emphysema/COPD, often single lung, idiopathic pulmonary fibrosis (IPF), and cystic fibrosis (CF). The primary goal of LTx is to improve prognosis, and this has been shown with CF and IPF, but the outcome in patients with COPD are less compelling. Guidelines for these common indications are:

- COPD: BODE (BMI, airways obstruction, dyspnoea, and exercise capacity), index of 7–10, or hospitalization with acute hypercapnia (pCO_2 >50mmHg (6.7kPa)), or pulmonary hypertension despite O_2 therapy, or FEV_1 <20% and DLCO (diffusing capacity of the lung for carbon monoxide) <20%, or homogenous distribution of emphysema.
- CF: FEV_1 <30% predicted, or a rapid decline in FEV_1; exacerbation requiring ITU, or frequent use of antibiotics; refractory/recurrent pneumothoraces; pulmonary hypertension, O_2-dependent respiratory failure; hypercapnia.
- IPF: DLCO <39% predicted; >10% fall in forced vital capacity (FVC) in 6 months; SpO_2 <88% in a 6-minute walk test; honeycombing on high-resolution CT (fibrosis score >2).

Contraindications

- Malignancy within 5 years
- Advanced major organ dysfunction (heart, kidney, liver)
- Poor compliance
- Poor social support
- Substance abuse
- Age—the prognosis is best in patients <50 years old
- Overt sepsis or hepatitis B/C, HIV infection
- Obesity (BMI >30)
- Other significant comorbidity.

Prognosis

The prognosis following LTx is poorer than following CTx (5.3 vs 10 years). A better outcome is seen in:

- Bilateral lung transplantation (compared with single lung)
- Younger recipients.

Postoperative management of lung transplant recipients

Following LTx, patients are managed in the ICU with close monitoring of graft function, immunosuppression, and for signs of infection (including CMV). Initial priorities include:

- Reverse isolation
- Early extubation (18–24 hours)

- Early mobilization
- Negative fluid balance.

Respiratory management

Maintain PaO_2 >80mmHg (10.7kPa) with the lowest inspired O_2 and PEEP possible.

Targets

- Tidal volume 6–8mL/kg
- PEEP 4–8cm/H_2O (note: a high PEEP may cause a deterioration in bronchial anastomotic healing, barotrauma, or over-inflation of the native lung in single LTx)
- Peak inspiratory pressure <30cmH_2O
- Pulmonary toilet 2-hourly
- Chest drain <15cm/H_2O suction
- Fibreoptic bronchoscopy if atelectasis/infiltration seen, or prior to extubation (to assess bronchial anastomosis and colour of distal bronchus).

Haemodynamic targets

- Central venous pressure (CVP) <10cmH_2O
- MAP >80mmHg
- Mean PAP <50mmHg
- Urine output >0.5mL/kg/hour
- Haematocrit >0.3.

Graft dysfunction

Early graft dysfunction occurs in ~20% of LTx. If oxygenation deteriorates, prompt investigation (including CXR, perfusion scintigraphy, echocardiography, and CT chest) should be carried out looking for the precipitating cause. Causes include:

- Pulmonary thrombosis/stenosis
- Pulmonary hypertension
- Mediastinal shift in single LTx/COPD
- Re-implant response (reperfusion injury caused by endothelial dysfunction, leading to pulmonary hypertension, pulmonary oedema, and respiratory failure).

LTx rejection

Acute rejection is characterized by perivascular mononuclear cell infiltrates, whereas chronic rejection is manifest by fibrous scarring, involving the bronchioles and sometimes associated with accelerated fibrointimal changes affecting pulmonary arteries and veins (Table 22.2). Infection and LTx rejection often occur together and can be confused histologically. For that reason, infection needs to be rigorously excluded for the accurate and reproducible interpretation of pulmonary allograft biopsies.

Investigations performed to identify LTx rejection include:

- CXR: performed twice daily for the first week, daily for the second week, then twice weekly. Ill-defined peri-hilar and lower zone nodules and septal lines may raise the suspicion of rejection, although a normal appearance does not exclude an episode of rejection.
- Spirometry: daily pulmonary function tests (PFTs) using a hand-held spirometer, and formal PFTs at discharge and at 3, 6, and 12 months. A >5% reduction in FEV_1 or VC may be suggestive of rejection.

- Transbronchial lung biopsy (TBLB): routinely performed using fluoroscopy at 10 days post LTx, at discharge, and at 3, 6, and 12 months. In cases of suspected rejection, biopsies are taken from each lung lobe showing abnormality on CXR.
- Bronchoalveolar lavage: 50mL aliquots of normal saline administered into infiltrated lobes and recovered by low suction into traps.

Immunosuppression

The majority of lung transplant centres now employ an immunosuppressive strategy that uses a combination of tacrolimus and mycophenolate, with a reducing dose of corticosteroids.

Infection

Infection is very common after lung transplantation due to denervation, bronchial anastomosis, impaired mucociliary function, immunosuppression, and bronchiolitis obliterans occurring as a chronic rejection. As such, bacterial, fungal, viral (particularly cytomegalovirus (CMV)) and protozoal (*Pneumocystis jirovecii* and toxoplasma) infections are a common cause of morbidity and mortality in the early postoperative period. CMV mismatched donors and recipients should be avoided where possible. Prophylaxis for infection should be adopted according to local protocol.

Table 22.2 Revised working formulation for classification and grading of pulmonary allograft rejection. 'R' denotes revised grade to avoid confusion with 1996 scheme

A: Acute rejection
Grade 0—non
Grade 1—minimal
Grade 2—mild
Grade 3—moderate
Grade 4—Severe
B: Airway inflammation
Grade 0—none
Grade 1R—low grade
Grade 2R—high grade
Grade X—ungradeable
C: Chronic airway rejection—obliterative bronchiolitis
0—absent
1—present
D: Chronic vascular rejection—accelerated graft vascular sclerosis

Reproduced from *The Journal of Heart and Lung Transplantation*, 26, 12, Stewart, S., et al, Revision of the 1996 Working Formulation for the Standardization of Nomenclature in the Diagnosis of Lung Rejection, pp.1229–1242, Copyright 2007, with permission from International Society for Heart and Lung Transplantation, and Elsevier.

Further reading

Orens JB, Estenne M, Arcasoy S, Conte JV, Corris P, Egan JJ, et al. International guidelines for the selection of lung transplant candidates: 2006 update. *J Heart Lung Transplant* 2006;25:745–55.

Heart–lung transplantation

The first successful heart–lung transplant was performed in 1981 by Dr Bruce Reitz at Stanford Hospital. The number of procedures reported to be performed worldwide is declining, with 50% of centres performing only one such transplant per year.

The primary indications for heart–lung transplantation are:
- Congenital heart disease (39%)
- Primary pulmonary hypertension (25%)
- CF (14%).

The procedure

The donor heart and lungs are harvested with minimal handling, with the heart flushed with cold cardioplegia solution, and the lungs with modified Collins solution.

Using CPB, the recipient's heart and lungs are removed whilst care is taken to preserve the phrenic nerves and to avoid postoperative bleeding complications from the bronchial artery circulation. The donor heart and lungs are inserted in the anastomotic order: trachea, right atrium, aorta. Care should be taken to keep the donor trachea as short as possible because of the limited vascularity of the area.

Prognosis

Although the prognosis has improved in recent years, the 1-year mortality is ~28%, and around half of patients are dead at 3 years. However, patients surviving the first year have an average life expectancy of nearly 10 years.

Immunosuppression

The calcineurin inhibitors (CNIs) ciclosporin and tacrolimus are the corner-stone of immunosuppressive regimens. Traditionally, either is used in combination with corticosteroids and an antiproliferative agent (mycophenolate or azathioprine). The use of induction therapy may delay the introduction of a CNI and reduce the incidence of perioperative renal dysfunction. Tacrolimus is thought to be somewhat more effective than ciclosporin, and mycophenolate has been shown to provide more effective prophylaxis against acute rejection compared with azathioprine. The combination of tacrolimus, mycophenolate, and corticosteroids may therefore be considered to be the most effective form of maintenance immunosuppression at least for the first 6–12 months after transplantation.

Calcineurin inhibitors

Ciclosporin (cyclosporine)

- Commenced when haemodynamics are stable, without evidence of hepatic or renal failure.
- Metabolized via cytochrome P450 pathway
- Starting dose: 4mg/kg/day orally or 1.5mg/kg/day IV in two divided doses (the IV dose is approximately a third of the oral dose).
- Subsequent dose depends on blood levels and renal function, and can be measured in two ways: C_0—trough level, or C_2—2 hours post dose.
- Target C_0 levels:
  - 300–400mcg/L for the first 4 weeks
  - 200–250mcg/L from 4 weeks to 6 months
  - 150–200mcg/L from 6 months to 1 year
  - 100–150mcg/L after 1 year.

Tacrolimus

- CNI
- 0.15–0.3mg/kg/day orally.

Antiproliferative immunosuppressants

Mycophenolate mofetil (MMF)

- As soon as the patient is able to take oral medications, MMF is commenced at a dose of 1.5g twice a day.
- Adjusted to mitigate side effects.

Azathioprine

- Day 0: 4mg/kg IV at induction
- Postoperatively: 2mg/kg/day as a single dose if white cell count >4
- Discontinued when MMF commenced.

Corticosteroids

- Intraoperative: 1g methylprednisolone at release of cross-clamp
- Days 1 and 2: 125mg methylprednisolone IV 12-hourly then oral prednisolone 60mg/day decreasing by 5mg each day and then stopped
- Thereafter, steroids given for acute rejection.

Target of rapamycin inhibitors

Sirolimus and everolimus

- Similar efficacy in prophylaxis against acute rejection as MMF.
- Limited use due to adverse effects:
  - Impaired wound healing
  - Pericardial effusions
  - Bacterial and fungal infections
  - GI effects
  - Pneumonitis (sirolimus)
  - Potentiates CNI nephrotoxicity
  - Drug interactions (cytochrome P450 pathway).

Induction therapy

Many centres use a form of induction therapy with an anti-T-cell antibody to provide additional immunosuppression during the early perioperative period, lower rates of acute rejection, possible host hyporesponsiveness to alloantigen, and renal protection by allowing the delayed introduction of the CNIs. Agents that have been used for this purpose include:

- Monomurab-CD3 (OKT3)
- Antithymocyte globulin (ATG)
- Basiliximab and daclizumab (monoclonal antibodies to the IL-2 receptor)
- Alemtuzumab (CAMPATH-1H)—humanized antibody against CD52. Profoundly depletes lymphocytes. Used in kidney transplantation; however, there is limited data in heart transplantation and there has been concern about potential cardiac toxicity.

Acute cardiology

Out-of-hospital cardiac arrest

Introduction

Cardiovascular disease is the leading cause of death in the developed world. There is a wide variation in the reported incidence and outcome of patients who have out-of-hospital cardiac arrest (OOHCA). It is unfortunately a common event with a high mortality, and survival rate to discharge home is typically <10%. The most common cause for adult cardiac arrest is acute coronary syndrome (ACS), however it is important to eliminate other potential causes and treat them appropriately.

Principles of management

- Effective cardiopulmonary resuscitation (CPR) with minimal interruption
- Optimize oxygenation
- Early defibrillation
- Appropriate drug treatment.

During circulatory arrest, organ injury can result from hypoxia, which is further exacerbated by reperfusion injury once return of spontaneous circulation (ROSC) is established. This insult can result in systemic inflammatory response syndrome (SIRS) and subsequent multiorgan failure (MOF). Early, aggressive management of these patients has potential to significantly influence their outcome and neurological status.

Post-cardiac care bundle (AHA guidelines)

1. Early coronary reperfusion

Early PCI is superior to thrombolysis with lower stroke, death, and reinfarction rates.

2. Hemodynamic optimization

Following cardiac arrest there is often a period of transient myocardial dysfunction; hypotension, reduced CO, frequent arrhythmias, and impaired contractility. Treatment includes:

- IABP may augment the failing myocardium by both offloading the heart and increasing coronary perfusion
- Inotropic/vasopressor support
- Invasive cardiac monitoring.

3. Control of ventilation

Management should aim to avoid ALI:

- Aim for normocarbia and oxygen saturation 94–98%
- Lung protective ventilation strategies:
  - Tidal volumes 6mL/kg
  - Use of PEEP
  - FiO_2 <60%
  - Permissive hypercapnia with plateau pressures <30cmH$_2$O.

4. Blood glucose control

Blood glucose should be kept within 6–10mmol/L.

5. Treatment of seizures

Seizures are common following hypoxic neurological insult:

* Insufficient evidence for prophylactic treatment.
* Tonic clonic seizures treated with phenytoin/sodium valproate/ benzodiazepines.
* Myoclonus can be treated with clonazepam.
* The use of EEG monitoring allows for identification of subclinical seizures, or seizure activity in paralysed patients.

6. Temperature control

Pyrexia is common in the 48 hours following cardiac arrest; poor neurological outcome has been associated with temperatures of 38°C and above.

Therapeutic hypothermia

There is increasing interest in the use of therapeutic hypothermia following OOHCA. Two landmark randomized control trials (RCTs) looked at the effect of cooling patients following VF arrest. Both trials demonstrated improvement in anoxic neurological injury, relating to improved functional outcomes and reduced mortality.

The International Liaison Committee on Resuscitation (ILCOR) recommends the use of therapeutic hypothermia in patients who have ROSC though remain comatose following OOHCA regardless of initial presenting rhythm.

Indications for therapeutic hypothermia

Patients accepted for ICU treatment directly or via the catheter lab with following features:

* OOHCA with ROSC regardless of presenting rhythm
* Comatose at the initial point of treatment with GCS score <9
* Cerebral irritation following ROSC requiring intubation
* No other known cause of coma (e.g. metabolic, trauma)
* No coma state *prior* to arrest
* No terminal illness
* Not pregnant (request HCG test if <50 years)
* Not haemodynamically unstable, e.g. high dose of inotropic support
* No severe respiratory compromise.

Due to the adverse physiological effects of cooling, it is important to assess the risk of benefit versus harm on an individual basis.

Temperature monitoring (in order of preference)

* PAFC
* Bladder
* Rectal
* Oesophageal
* Do not use tympanic probe for temperature monitoring—this is inaccurate.

Protocol for therapeutic hypothermia

See Fig. 23.1.

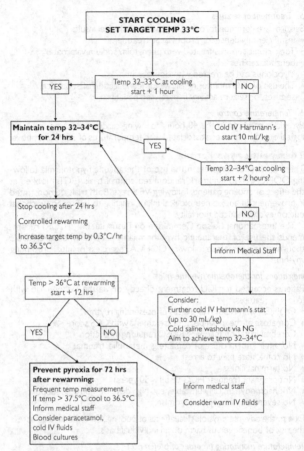

Figure 23.1 (a) and (b) An example of a protocol for therapeutic hypothermia. Reproduced with kind permission from Jorg Prinzlin and Kenneth McKinlay, Copyright Golden Jubilee National Hospital.

Further reading

Intensive Care Society (ICS), UK. *Standards for the Management of Patients After Cardiac Arrest.* <http://www.ics.ac.uk/ics-homepage/guidelines-standards/>.

Endocarditis

Introduction

Endocarditis is inflammation of the endocardium, which may or may not include the heart valves. Despite advances in medicine over the last 30 years neither the incidence nor mortality of the condition has changed. However, both the predisposing factors and causative agents have altered. Previously considered a disease of the young with rheumatic heart disease, now this condition is associated with older patients following invasive procedures with or without prosthetic heart valves.

Predisposing factors

- Male > female
- Increasing age
- IV drug abuse
- Valve prostheses
- Degenerative valve sclerosis
- Multiple invasive procedures
- Chronic haemodialysis
- Diabetes
- Intravascular devices.

Microbiology

85% of cases are blood culture positive for the following typical bacteria:

- *Staphylococcus aureus*: commonest causative bacteria, coagulase negative *Staphylococcus* is frequently associated with prosthetic valve endocarditis (PVE)
- *Streptococcus; S. sangius, S. mitis, S. salivarius, S. mutans*, and *Gemella morbillorum*. Infection with *S. milleri* and *S. anginosus* is associated with abscess formation and disseminated disease
- *Enterococcus; E. faecalis, E. faecium, E. durans*.

Blood cultures are frequently negative with the following organisms:

- Variant *Streptococcus*
- Gram-negative bacilli
- HACEK group (*Haemophilus, Actinobacillus, Cardiobacterium, Eikenella, Kingella*)
- *Brucella*, and fungi.

Up to 5% of cases are the result of *Coxiella burnetii* (Q fever), *Bartonella, Legionella, Mycoplasma*, and *Chlamydia*. These organisms will always have negative blood cultures and can only be identified with serology and cell culture.

Common presenting features

- New regurgitant murmur
- Embolic event—30% patients present with brain, lung, or spleen infarction
- Fever, signs of sepsis, pyrexia of unknown origin (PUO).

Additional features
- Splinter haemorrhages (particularly on nail beds)
- Janeway lesions (painless macular erythematous lesions)
- Roth spots (retinal haemorrhages)
- Osler's nodes (painful nodules on digits)
- Rigors, fatigue, anaemia, night sweats, microscopic haematuria.

Diagnosis
The Duke criteria for diagnosis of infective endocarditis require 2 major or 1 major and 3 minor or 5 minors:

Major criteria
- Positive blood cultures: either typical organism in 2 sets, or persistently positive blood cultures (3+ sets >12 hours apart), or single positive blood culture for Q fever/phase 1 IgG antibody titre > 1:800.
- Endocardium involvement: echocardiogram evidence of vegetation/abscesses or new valvular incompetence.

Minor criteria
- Predisposing factors
- Pyrexia > 38°C
- Positive blood cultures
- Echocardiogram that do not meet major criteria
- Vascular or immunological signs.

Investigations
- *Blood cultures*: at least 3 sets taken 30 minutes apart from separate sites.
- *Echocardiogram*: TTE is first line in all patients; TOE has a higher sensitivity and specificity and is indicated in patients with a high suspicion of infective endocarditis (IE) despite a negative TTE and in all patients who have a positive TTE (abscess/vegetations visualized). In patients in whom a high suspicion remains despite previously negative findings should be rescanned 7–10 days later.
- *Urinalysis*: microscopic haematuria.
- *CXR*: cardiomegaly.
- *ECG*: conduction abnormalities, typically 1st-degree heart block.
- *Blood tests*: normochromic, normocytic anaemia, leukopenia, raised ESR and CRP.

Management
Early antibiotic therapy has been shown to reduce mortality.
Empirical therapy for native valves with acute presentation:
- Flucloxacillin 8–12g/day in 4–6 doses with gentamycin 1mg/kg/day three times a day.
- In penicillin allergic patients: vancomycin 1g/12 hours, and gentamycin 1mg/kg/day three times a day.

Subacute presentation:
- Penicillin 7.2g in 6 divided doses with gentamycin 1mg/kg/day three times a day, or
- Amoxicillin 12g/day in 6 divided doses (more activity against HACEK organisms).

Prosthetic valves
- Vancomycin and gentamycin doses as previously with the addition of rifampicin 600–1200mg/day in two oral doses.

Once organism is isolated therapy should be directed in accordance with microbiological advice.

Early surgery prevents progressive heart failure and valvular destruction; however it also carries a higher mortality risk. The indications for surgery are:
- Uncontrolled infection despite treatment
- Prevention of emboli
- Heart failure.

Prophylaxis
Certain patients are considered at a higher risk of developing endocarditis:
- Patients with prosthetic valves/material for cardiac valve repair
- Patients with previous infective endocarditis
- Structural congenital heart disease—not including isolated atrial septal defect, repaired ventricular septal defect, or patent ductus arteriosus
- Hypertrophic cardiomyopathy
- Acquired valve heart disease (stenosis/incompetence).

Prophylactic antibiotics:
- No longer indicated for all dental or non-dental procedures as the risk of anaphylaxis outweighs the benefit of use.
- Advice is given regarding recognizing symptoms, good oral hygiene, and avoidance of potential causative procedures.
- However, if a high risk patient has an infection which requires antibiotics, and is undergoing GU/GI surgery at the site of the infection then antibiotics given should cover organisms causative for IE.

Prognosis is dependent on four features:
- *Patient factors*: elderly, PVE, coexisting disease – respiratory, renal, cardiac, or IDDM.
- *Infective organism*: fungi, *Staphylococcus aureus*, and Gram-negative bacilli all have poorer outcomes.
- *Complications* of IE are heart or renal failure, CVA, and septic shock.
- *Echocardiogram* evidence of pulmonary hypertension, severe valvular incompetence, raised diastolic pressure and reduced LV ejection fraction.

Further reading
Habib G, Hoen B, Tornos P, Thuny F, Prendergast B, Vilacosta I, et al. Guidelines on the prevention, diagnosis, and treatment of infective endocarditis (new version 2009): the Task Force on the Prevention, Diagnosis, and Treatment of Infective Endocarditis of the European Society of Cardiology (ESC). *Eur Heart J* 2009;30:2369–413.

Aortic dissection

Introduction

Separation of the intima and media layers of the aortic wall results in the formation of both false and true lumens. Blood within the false lumen can then sequestrate and result in the dissection extending and potentially rupturing.

Risk factors

- Male > female
- 50–70 years
- Hypertension, smoking, and hyperlipidaemia.

Causes

- Congenital: Marfan's syndrome, Ehler–Danlos syndrome, Turner's syndrome
- Degenerative: age >60
- Atherosclerotic: hypertension, smoking, and hyperlipidaemia are all risk factors
- Inflammatory: Takayasu's disease, Behçet's disease, giant cell arteritis, rheumatoid arthritis, and Ormond's disease
- Traumatic: deceleration injury—road traffic collision, fall from height
- Surgical/iatrogenic: cross-clamp or aortic cannula placement, angiography, or angioplasty
- Toxic: bacterial and fungal aortitis
- Drugs: cocaine and amphetamine use
- Pregnancy.

Classification

See Fig. 23.2.

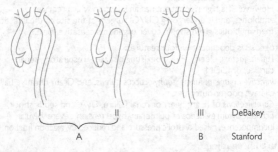

Figure 23.2 Classification of aortic dissection. Adapted from *The Annals of Thoracic Surgery*, 10, 3, Daily PO, Trueblood HW, Stinson EB, Wuerflein RD, Shumway NE, Management of acute aortic dissections, pp. 237–247. Copyright 1970, with permission from The Society of Thoracic Surgeons, and from *Journal of Thoracic Cardiovascular Surgery*, 49, DeBakey ME et al., Surgical management of dissecting aneurysms of the aorta, pp. 130–149. Copyright Elsevier 1965.

Stanford[1]

- Type A: the ascending aorta is involved in the dissection.
- Type B: no involvement of the ascending aorta.

DeBakey (further subdivides the dissection)[2]

- Type I the whole aorta is involved.
- Type II only the ascending aorta is involved.
- Type III only the descending aorta is involved in the dissection.

A new classification includes the aetiology of the dissection (Table 23.1).

Table 23.1 European Society of Cardiology classification of aortic dissection

Class 1	Classical aortic dissection
Class 2	Intramural haematoma/haemorrhage
Class 3	Subtle, discrete aortic dissection
Class 4	Plaque rupture/ulceration
Class 5	Traumatic/iatrogenic aortic dissection

Reproduced from Erbel R. et al., 'Diagnosis and management of aortic dissection: Task Force on Aortic Dissection, European Society of Cardiology', *European Heart Journal*, 2001, 22, 18, pp. 1642–1681, by permission of the European Society of Cardiology.

Presentation

- Abrupt onset of severe chest pain, typically radiating through to back.
- Pain often described as sharp, tearing, ripping, or stabbing.
- Associated syncope, cardiac failure, cardiac tamponade, aortic regurgitation, hypo/hypertension.
- Depending on the anatomy of the extension, aortic root occlusion can occur, affecting arms/legs (20%), renal (15%), brain (5%), cardiac (10%), and bowel (3%).

Diagnosis

Early diagnosis requires good history taking and a high index of suspicion in patients with risk factors.

- *ECG*: eliminate acute MI as the diagnosis. Extension of the dissection involving the coronary ostia may present as ischaemia on the ECG.
- *CXR*: mediastinal widening, cardiomegaly, aortic knuckles, pleural capping, deviation of trachea to right, and blunted costophrenic angles secondary to haemothorax.
- *CT*: high sensitivity and specificity of dissection, rapid test, and able to establish the extent of the lesion.
- *MRI*: highest sensitivity and specificity for diagnosis, also allows for functional assessment of aortic valve and left ventricle. May be impractical in critically ill patient.

1 Reprinted from *The Annals of Thoracic Surgery*, 10, 3, Daily PO, Trueblood HW, Stinson EB, Wuerflein RD, Shumway NE, Management of acute aortic dissections, pp. 237–247. Copyright 1970, with permission from The Society of Thoracic Surgeons.

2 This classification was published in *Journal of Thoracic Cardiovascular Surgery*, 49, DeBakey ME et al., Surgical management of dissecting aneurysms of the aorta, pp. 130–149. Copyright Elsevier 1965.

- *TOE*: allows for real time assessment of dissection, involvement of the aortic valve, degree of regurgitation, and left ventricular cardiac function can be assessed.
- *Aortography*: previously considered the gold standard, though inappropriate in unstable patient.

Differential diagnosis

- ACS
- Aortic regurgitation
- Aortic aneurysm without dissection
- Pericarditis
- PE
- Pleurisy.

Management

Type A aortic dissection

- Requires surgical intervention and has a higher mortality compared to type B (60% vs 10%).
- Mortality increases 1–2% per hour in the untreated acute ascending aorta dissections in the first 48 hours.

Type B aortic dissection

- Medical therapy is aimed at reducing hypertension.
- No evidence to suggest an improved survival in patients who have a surgical repair of type B aortic dissections.
- Surgery or interventional radiology may be considered in this group if the dissection is causing organ ischaemia.

Initial management

Strategy should be to prevent further extension of the dissection and vessel rupture:

- A, B, C.
- Tight BP control: IV labetalol to maintain systolic BP 80–100mmHg. Sodium nitroprusside (SNP), GTN and hydralazine are alternatives.
- Reduce LV contractility without comprising coronary perfusion.
- Adequate analgesia.
- IV access, cross-match, full blood count, coagulation, U&Es, lactate.
- Establish invasive monitoring—arterial line ideally placed in left radial artery as innominate artery may be involved in dissection, affecting right radial readings.

Conduct of anaesthesia

- Maintain haemodynamic stability.
- Type B dissections—thoracotomy incisions require double-lumen tube placement, usually left.
- Depending on position of aortic clamp patients are at risk of bowel or renal ischaemia and anterior spinal artery syndrome/paralysis.
- Meticulous review of urine output, metabolic status, and coagulation is important to anticipate any complications.
- TOE can help guide surgical decision-making.
- CPB—it may be necessary to establish CPB rapidly in a patient in extremis and femoral bypass can be established prior to sternotomy.

Deep hypothermic circulatory arrest (DHCA)

CPB allows for the maintenance of organ perfusion following cardioplegia induced cardiac arrest. Complete circulatory arrest can be advantageous in aortic surgery, providing improved operating conditions and reducing basal metabolic rate (BMR) and organ ischaemia. By reducing the body temperature to 18–20°C prolongation of the CPB and aortic cross-clamp times are possible. Periods of up to 30 minutes of DHCA are tolerated without significant neurological dysfunction; longer durations are linked to a sharp increase in neurological injury and poorer outcome.

It is possible to selectively perfuse the cerebral circulation, using retrograde cerebral perfusion or selective antegrade cerebral perfusion. By using these methods DHCA can be prolonged safely.

Postoperative care

- Establish normothermia.
- Correct any coagulopathy and acidosis.
- Maintain MAP ~65mmHg for at least the first 4 hours following the operation and if no significant bleeding noted increase the MAP ~75mmHg.
- Careful fluid balance, risk of cerebral oedema formation, may require mannitol or frusemide therapy.
- Keep the patient ventilated and sedated initially, once haemodynamically stable for >12 hours and no signs of bleeding, wean patients and assess neurological status.

Further reading

Erbel R, Alfonso F, Boileau C, Dirsch O, Eber B, Haverich A, et al. Diagnosis and management of aortic dissection. Eur Heart J 2001;22:1642–81.

Hebballi R, Swanevelder J. Diagnosis and management of aortic dissection. CEACCP 2009;9:14–18.

Part 4

Treatments and procedures

Central venous cannulation, pulmonary artery catheter, and minimally invasive cardiac output monitoring

Central venous cannulation

Indications
- Measurement of central venous pressure (CVP)
- If peripheral venous access is difficult to establish
- Administration of drugs which cannot be given peripherally. Administration of TPN and other hypertonic solutions
- Siting of PAFC
- Transvenous cardiac pacing
- Renal replacement therapy.

Preventing complications
15% of patients with central venous catheters have a complication.
- Use standard Seldinger wire technique.
- Ultrasound technique reduces risk of arterial puncture and pneumothorax. Particularly useful in internal jugular vein (IJV) cannulation.
- Choose multilumen catheters to avoid multiple cannulations.
- Get experienced help if more than 3 cannulation attempts: (risk ↑× 6).
- Prevent air embolism: occlude lumina during insertion, use head-down position (may not be tolerated with poor cardiac function).
- Arterial puncture? Check pressure trace or compare blood sample to ABG.
- Arrhythmias: check ECG whilst advancing Seldinger wire or catheter.
- Perforation: usually delayed complication due to erosion of vessel wall. Risk of damaging veins (stiff PAC introducer) and endocardium (PAC).
- Central venous thrombosis: ↑ risk in IJV, femoral vein, and large catheters.
- Pneumothorax: ↑ risk with hyperinflation (large TV, PEEP, chronic obstructive airways disease). If suspected do not attempt contralateral IJV/subclavian vein (SCV) cannulation.

Preventing infection
- Risk of bloodstream infection is 3–8%.
- Mechanism of catheter infection:
  - <15 days: tip colonization with skin organisms via ext. tract.
  - >15 days: contamination of catheter, organisms via int. lumen.
- Maximal precautions: hat, mask, gown, gloves, large sterile drapes. Skin antisepsis with chlorhexidine is significantly superior.
- Use Teflon or polyurethane catheters.
- Antimicrobial catheters ↓ infection risk but may ↑ antibiotic resistance. Consider if infection rate is high despite preventative measures. Antibiotic ointments at catheter site ↑ resistance and fungal infections.
- Give lipids (TPN, propofol) via dedicated lumina.
- Changing of CVC over guidewires ↑ infection risk.
- Scheduled replacement of CVC does not reduce infection risk.
- Remove CVC as soon as not required.

Central vein routes

In cardiothoracic patients IJV, SCV, and femoral veins are commonly used.

Internal jugular cannulation

- Easily accessible and high success rate.
- Low complication rate with landmark technique, best with ultrasound.
- Safer than SCV approach in deranged coagulation. External pressure on punctured carotid artery possible.
- Right IJV preferred because of straight access into SVC. Low left-sided approach carries risk of thoracic duct damage (chylothorax).
- May be less comfortable for awake patients than subclavian route.
- Awake patient: insertion with LA infiltration or superficial cervical plexus block.
- Head-down tilt to increase venous filling and prevent air embolus.
- Venous thrombosis risk approximately 4× that of the SCV.
- High approach in neck reduces risk of pneumo/haemothorax.

Subclavian vein cannulation

- More comfortable for patient
- Least risk of infection
- Ultrasound less useful as vein is more difficult to visualize
- Risk ↑ of pneumothorax; arterial puncture—compression difficult.

Femoral vein cannulation

- Arterial puncture: easily compressible
- No risk of pneumothorax
- Indicated in SVC obstruction
- Difficult to mobilize patients
- ↑ risk of infection in patients with BMI >28
- ↑ risk of thrombosis (up to 21%).

Central line tip position

- To avoid vessel wall erosion and pericardial tamponade catheter tip must lie outside the RA and parallel to the SVC just above the pericardial inflection (CXR: the carina is the landmark just above this).
- Innominate vein position: thrombosis risk with inotropes/irritant drugs.
- Right-sided catheters should be sited above the carina.
- Left-sided catheters may need to be positioned distal to the carina to avoid the tip abutting on SVC wall.
- CVC tip changes 2–3cm with respiration, arm, and torso position.
- If in doubt about the correct length, insert a longer catheter deep and withdraw after CXR.

Pulmonary artery catheter

There is controversy on safety and clinical benefit of the PAC. It continues to be used in CICU as the only device that can assess intrathoracic pressures, CO, and SvO_2 simultaneously. Standard PAC features: 10cm markings, proximal lumen for CVP and IV fluids, distal lumen for PAWP, balloon lumen and thermistor for CO measurement near the tip, and fibreoptic bundles for continuous SvO_2 measurement. See Table 24.1.

Indication

- Monitoring of SvO_2, cardiac pressures, CO, and derived data: trends more useful than single values
- Differentiation of causes of shock states
- Assessment of pulmonary hypertension
- Differentiation of high- versus low-pressure pulmonary oedema
- Aspiration of air emboli.

Contraindications

- Tricuspid or pulmonary valve mechanical prosthesis or endocarditis
- Right heart mass (thrombus/tumour).

Insertion

- Insert PAFC introducer. Preferred routes: right IJV, left SCV (no acute angle to enter SVC); femoral veins can be difficult (in enlarged RV).
- Full-barrier asepsis for insertion. Check balloon, pre-fill other lumina. Inside sterile plastic sleeve catheter can be freely handled.
- Attach transducer to distal lumen. Observe pressure changes as catheter is advanced. Calibrate (usually automatic), reference (as for CVP) and zero prior measurements. Avoid dampening (bubbles)—check with rapid flush test.
- Patient supine or head-up. Curved catheter tip may help positioning (RIJ: curve to L shoulder, in RV turn ¼ clockwise to ease tip into PA).
- In RA inflate the balloon gently (1mL/sec) and 'float' from the RV into PA. Max. filling of balloon 1.5mL. As the balloon occludes a PA vessel the pressure trace changes (Fig. 24.1). This is the PAWP.
- Deflate the balloon and ensure PA trace becomes visible again. If permanent wedging occurs, gently withdraw the catheter.
- In-between PAWP measurement, ensure balloon stays deflated to avoid PA damage and infarction. Monitor PAP trace continuously.
- CXR: tip position below level of left atrium (only 60% of catheters).
- Aim to remove catheter within 72 hours to reduce complications.

Difficulties floating the catheter

- In RA or RV dilation, severe TR, very poor RV function:
  - Optimize patient position: head up and slightly towards the right side puts pulmonary valve at the highest level. When the catheter is in the RV outflow tract (PVCs), pause ventilator in inspiration and advance catheter into PA.
- Consider fluoroscopy.

Table 24. 1 Cardiac pressures related to PAC length and position (RIJ approach)

Position	Length (cm)	Pressure (mmHg)
RA	20–25	0–8/0–8
RV	30–35	15–30/3–8
PA	40–45	15–30/4–12
PA wedge	45–55	2–15

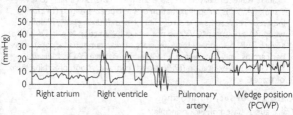

Pressure tracings during pulmonary artery catheterization

Figure 24.1 PAC waveform changes on insertion. SVC /RA: = CVP waveform; RV trace: after crossing TV, steady increase in diastolic pressure; PAP trace: after crossing PV, sudden rise in diastolic pressure with steady fall in baseline; PAWP: similar to CVP trace. Reproduced from Punit S. Ramrakha and Kevin P. Moore, *Oxford Handbook of Acute Medicine* 2nd Edition, 2004, figure in chapter 16, p. 879, with permission from Oxford University Press.

Complications

- Mechanical and infective complications as with central venous access.
- Arrhythmia: usually PVCs, short-lived VT. Significant VT/VF in <1%. Transient right bundle branch block (BBB) in 5% (risk of 3rd-degree heart block with pre-existing left BBB).
- Infection (↑ risk after day 3).
- Coiling/knotting: suspect if >20cm advanced into the RV without waveform changes. Withdraw slowly to avoid knotting. Get experienced help, consider fluoroscopy, interventional radiology.
- Damage to valves, myocardium.
- Rupture/damage to PA: rare (~1% but 50% fatal). Risk ↑: pulmonary hypertension, >60 years, anticoagulation. Signs: sudden haemoptysis after inflation of PAC balloon. Management: position bleeding side down, lung isolation with DLT, PEEP, embolization or lobectomy.
- Pulmonary infarction: (<7%) Cause: migration of PAC or thrombi.
- PAC not in zone 3; suspect if: mean PAWP >mean pulmonary artery diastolic pressure (PADP), PAP trace swings ++ with respiration.

Difficulties determining the PAC position

- Large v waves may make it difficult to differentiate PA trace and PCWP. Look for subtle waveform differences (loss of the PA dicrotic notch) or compare distal blood sample with and without balloon inflation (PAWP = SvO_2, PAP = SaO_2).
- Overwedging: wedge pressure trace rises excessively, no pulsatile trace, balloon volume less than half the maximum.

Cardiac pressures

- PAP: approx. 1/5 of systemic pressures.
- PAWP: pressure at the distal catheter tip as balloon occludes a PA branch. Reflects delayed pressure changes in the LA (similar to CVP trace). PAWP is an approximation of the true LV preload (LVEDV), indirectly represents myocardial fibre length (Starling law). Helpful when RA pressures (CVP) do not reflect LV function, e.g. in LV failure, severe BBB, pulmonary hypertension, cardiac tamponade, constrictive pericarditis, valvular disease. ~1–4mmHg less than PADP. Measure PAWP at end-expiration (IPPV: trough of trace, spont. breathing: peak of trace).

Cardiac output monitoring

Calculations based on Fick principle:

- *Intermittent:* 10mL cold fluid boluses into RA, blood temperature measured by thermistor at tip, use average from 3–4 measurements.
- *Continuous CO (CCO):* pseudo-random cycles from RA heat element every 40–60 seconds registered by thermistor. Temperature–time-curve is inversely proportional to CO. Changes may lag up to 12 minutes.
- Pitfalls: large left-to-right shunt: overestimation of CO, large right-to-left shunt: underestimation of CO, severe TR: may over or underestimate CO.

Interpretation

(See Table 24.2.)

Table 24. 2 Haemodynamic parameters in relation to common disorders

	CO	PAWP	CVP	SVR
Cardiogenic	↓	↑	↑	↑
Vasodilatation	↑	↔/↓	↔/↓	↓
Hypovolaemia	↓	↓	↓	↑

- Cardiac tamponade: ↑ RA pressure on inspiration (Kussmaul sign), mean RA pressure = RVDP = PADP = PAWP.
- Cardiogenic pulmonary oedema: likely if PAWP >18–20mmHg (if colloid pressure and permeability normal).
- PAWP overestimates LVED pressure in mitral stenosis, PEEP ventilation, left atrial myoma, pulmonary hypertension.
- PAWP underestimates LVED pressure in non-compliant LV, LVED >25mmHg, aortic regurgitation.

Mixed venous oximetry

Indicates VO_2/DO_2 balance and adequacy of global circulation. High risk of poor tissue oxygenation if SvO_2 <40%. See Table 24.3.

Table 24. 3 Common causes of abnormal SvO_2

Low SvO_2		High SvO_2	
VO_2 ↑	DO_2 ↓	VO_2 ↓	DO_2 ↑
Shivering	Hb ↓	Sedation	Hb ↑
Stress/pain	FiO_2 ↓	Hypothermia	FiO_2 ↑
Hyperthermia	CO ↓	Muscle relaxation	CO ↑
Seizures		Sepsis (shunting)	
		Wedged PAC (artefact)	

Minimally invasive cardiac output monitoring

Several alternatives to the PAC are being used to assess cardiac function:

Pulse contour analysis

Area under the curve (AUC) of a central arterial pressure wave (PW) correlates with the stroke volume (SV) calculated from aortic compliance and pressures. These are estimated by mathematical modelling from peripheral arterial PW. Difficulties arise from the accuracy of determining the systolic part of arterial PW, estimating varying arterial compliance and quality of PW.

Pulse contour analysis with calibration

- Lithium indicator dilution (LiDCOplus):
- Calibration for SV: an arterial sensor measures the concentration of a lithium bolus. CO calculated from this. Recalibration ≤8 hours or in haemodynamic instability.
- Continuous mode: assumes changes in the arterial PW to reflect SV.
- Accuracy decreases with: AF, IABP, AV disease, quaternary muscle relaxants, severe hyponatraemia. The system should not be used in 1st trimester pregnancy, concurrent lithium therapy, body weight <40kg. Transpulmonary cold indicator dilution (PiCCO).
- Calibration for SV: cold saline injected into central vein. Temperature changes detected by a peripheral arterial sensor. Allows estimation of extra vascular lung water (EVLW). Needs frequent recalibration in haemodynamic instability.
- Continuous mode: analyses systolic AUC, shape of PW, aortic compliance and SVR calculated CO.
- Accuracy ↓ in cardiac shunt, severe AV disease, and IABP.

Non-calibrated pulse contour analysis (Vigileo™)

- No venous access or calibration required.
- Algorithm uses demographics, analysis of pulse pressure (~ to SV), SD of 2000 data points of arterial PW to estimate arterial compliance and calculate SV and CO.
- Accuracy ↓ with AR, severe peripheral arterial vasoconstriction. Not validated with concurrent use of IABP.

Thoracic bioimpedance measurement

- Thoracic electrodes emit and sense a small alternating current and relate it to the ECG. Baseline impedance reflects total thoracic fluid volume. The change in impedance over the cardiac cycle generates a waveform similar to the aortic flow curve and allows calculation of SV, CO, and myocardial contractility.
- Accuracy may be affected by pulmonary oedema and changes in PVR. Validity in critically ill and cardiac patients is uncertain.

Oesophageal Doppler

- Velocity of blood flow is proportional to frequency of reflected waves (Doppler shift). Probe is rotated for optimal velocity-time signals. Shape of waveform reflects peak velocity, LV preload, contractility, and afterload. Aortic cross-section area estimated from nomograms or measured by oesophageal probe. Calculation of SV and CO assumes flow through the ascending aorta stays constant.
- Accuracy ↓ by hypovolaemia, regional anaesthesia. Good correlation with PAC for CO. Better reflection of preload (end-diastolic volume) than PAWP.

Further reading

Funk DJ, Moretti EW, Gan TJ. Minimally invasive cardiac output monitoring in the perioperative setting. *Anesthes Analg* 2009;108:887–97.

NICE. *Guidance on the use of Ultrasound locating devices for placing central venous catheters*, Technology Appraisal Guidance No 49. London: National Institute for Clinical Excellence; 2002.

Practice Guidelines for Pulmonary Artery Catheterization, An updated Report by the American Society of Anesthesiologists Task Force of on Pulmonary Artery Catheterization. *Anaesthesiology* 2003;99:988–1014.

Taylor RW, Paligri AV. Central venous cannulation. *Crit Care Med* 2007;35:1390–6.

Airway management

Intubation

Indications for intubation

- Hypoxaemia
- Hypercapnia
- Exhaustion
- To reduce the work of breathing and oxygen consumption
- To protect the airway (reduced GCS score/impaired laryngeal reflexes)
- To treat or prevent obstructed airway
- To facilitate investigations/treatment or critical care transfer.

The decision to institute mechanical ventilation can be difficult. It should be undertaken as a treatment for respiratory failure or critical illness if:
- The patient had an acceptable premorbid quality of life
- There is a reversible cause for the deterioration
- NIV is inappropriate
- The patient consents to the treatment or has not expressed any prior wishes regarding treatment limitation.

Technique of endotracheal intubation

Equipment and preparation

- Assess the airway—anticipate difficult intubation where possible.
- Allocate roles to appropriate skilled personnel.
- Have a plan in place for failed intubation.
- Check suction and ventilator or anaesthetic machine.
- Ensure there is an alternative working oxygen supply available.
- Have available a bag/valve/mask, laryngoscope, airway adjuncts, and various ETTs.
- Attach monitoring to Association of Anaesthetists of Great Britain and Ireland (AAGBI) standards: pulse oximeter, non-invasive blood pressure (NIBP), and ECG. Airway gas analysis including end-tidal CO_2 and airway pressure monitoring should be available immediately after intubation.
- In critically ill patients, insert an arterial line if time permits.
- Establish IV access with fluid attached.
- Draw up and label drugs of choice and emergency drugs
- Check trolley tips or head of bed able to tilt down
- Optimize patient position: neck flexed about 35° and head extended 15°. A pillow is required

Technique

- Preoxygenate with 100% oxygen with a tight fitting face mask for 3–5 minutes. In emergencies four vital capacity breaths may be used.
- Administer a sleep dose of a preselected IV induction agent followed by either a dose of depolarizing muscle relaxant in a rapid-sequence intubation (RSI) or non-depolarizing muscle relaxant.
- For example: thiopentone 3–7mg/kg followed by suxamethonium 100mg.
- If cricoid pressure is being used in an RSI then this should be applied by a skilled operator before loss of consciousness.

- In critically ill patients, administer an inotrope/vasoconstrictor or vasoconstrictor prophylactically—do not wait for hypotension to develop.
- Once muscle relaxation is established, a curved blade is placed into the right-hand side of the mouth using the left-handed laryngoscope. It is passed over the surface of the tongue and the tip placed between the epiglottis and the base of the tongue.
- The laryngoscope is lifted in the direction of the handle to reveal the glottis and vocal cords.
- The ETT (usually size 8–9mm for a male and 7–8mm for a female) is then inserted under direct vision from the right side of the mouth between the vocal cords and into the trachea.
- The tracheal cuff should then be inflated until no leak is audible or to 30cmH$_2$O.

Confirmation of correct placement
- Bilateral chest wall movement
- Auscultation of both lung fields for breath sounds
- Presence of exhaled CO$_2$ on capnography.

Once tracheal intubation is confirmed, cricoid pressure can be removed and the ETT should be secured with a tie or tape. In the critical care setting a chest radiograph is taken to confirm tube position.

Tracheostomy

This section deals with elective insertion of temporary tracheostomies in critically ill patients.

Some indications are absolute:
- Airway protection (neurological dysfunction)
- Upper airway obstruction

Some indications are relative:
- Bronchial toilet
- Patient may be cared for in lower dependency area
- Patient is poorly tolerant of ETT.

Most tracheostomies are placed in patients who are undergoing, or are at risk of, prolonged mechanical ventilation.

Anecdotal advantages:
- Improved patient comfort
- Reduction in sedation requirement
- Improved mouth care
- Reduced dead space, tube resistance, and work of breathing
- Improved weaning and reduced ICU length of stay.

Two recent prospective randomized trials evaluating early vs late placement of tracheostomy did not demonstrate any significant advantages of early tracheostomy, but did confirm that a policy of early tracheostomy inevitably means additional procedures and procedural complications.

Types

Percutaneous versus surgical

Where the expertise exists, percutaneous tracheostomy is now the preferred procedure in ICU (it is at least equivalent, possibly with less wound infections).

Internal/external diameter

Nomenclature used by different manufacturers is confusing. There is a reasonable amount of variation in the ratio of internal to external diameter, and different tubes all of the same 'size' may have significantly different internal diameters. The smaller the internal diameter the higher the imposed work of breathing.

Inner cannula and cuffs

Tubes with inner cannulae are safer, especially in areas without airway expertise, but the internal diameter is necessarily reduced compared with external diameter.

In the critical care setting, cuffed tubes are customarily the initial choice, allowing airway protection and positive pressure ventilation. Cuff pressure should be 20–30cmH$_2$O, to reduce VAP without causing mucosal ischaemia.

Fenestrations

If bulbar function is intact and the patient has been weaned from respiratory support, fenestrated tubes allow airflow through the upper airways and therefore phonation and speaking. If the tube is not fenestrated, deflating the cuff serves a similar function.

Shape and size

There is no perfect tracheostomy tube that will have the correct intra-stomal length, intra-tracheal length, and angulation for every patient. Alternatives should therefore be available in order to avoid problems with the tube abutting the anterior or posterior wall, tube displacement, or tracheal erosion. Adjustable flange tubes may be useful, but have no inner cannula.

Performing a tracheostomy

For guidance on how to perform a tracheostomy, see the Intensive Care Society's guidance on standards for the care of an adult patient with a temporary tracheostomy (see ▢ Further reading, p. 271.

Complications of tracheostomies

Immediate
- Pneumothorax or pneumomediastinum
- Tracheo-oesophageal fistula
- Injury to great vessels or recurrent laryngeal nerves
- Bleeding, e.g. from divided thyroid isthmus.

Early
- Secretions and mucus plugging
- Dislodged tube, respiratory arrest
- Post obstructive pulmonary oedema (when tracheostomy is performed in a patient with longstanding upper airway obstruction).

Late
- Bleeding from tracheoinnominate fistula (can be torrential)
- Tracheal stenosis (from ischemia induced by a cuffed tracheostomy tube)
- Tracheo-oesophageal fistula
- Tracheocutaneous fistula
- Cosmetic deformity.

Practical tracheostomy issues

Changing a tracheostomy

There is little evidence to guide practice. Facilities to reintubate via oral route should be immediately available.
- There is usually a defined stoma after 10 days.
- First elective change is best undertaken between 7 and 10 days. Avoid changes <72 hours after tracheostomy unless absolutely necessary.
- Railroad new tube over a fibreoptic scope (direct vision) or paediatric ETT (may be used to ventilate) or a suction catheter.

Tracheostomy emergencies

The main life-threatening complications associated with a tracheostomy are blockage, dislodgement, and bleeding (see Fig. 25.1).

Blockage and displacement

A blocked or displaced tracheostomy tube presents with respiratory diffi-culty. A partly dislodged tracheostomy tube is just as dangerous, if not more dangerous, as a completely removed tracheostomy tube.

- Tracheostomy tubes may become dislodged or displaced when a ventilated patient is turned, or moved from their bed to a trolley.
- Restless or agitated patients may pull at their tracheostomy tubes, or ventilator tubing attached to the tracheostomy.

Action

- Don't panic!
- Call for help—senior medical and nursing staff, other AHPs with tracheostomy care skills (e.g. physiotherapist).
- Reassure patient.
- Assess patency of airway (A) and patient's breathing (B). Is air passing through the tracheostomy tube or stoma? Is the patient breathing via mouth or nose?
- Check capnography and oxygen saturation with a pulse oximeter.
- *If airway is not patent, it must be cleared immediately.*
- If the blocked tracheostomy tube has an inner lumen, remove the inner lumen and ventilate through the outer lumen.
- If a single-lumen tracheostomy tube is blocked or displaced, obstructing the airway, remove it to ventilate through the stoma or the mouth/nose.
- Once removed, only experienced staff should attempt to re-insert a tracheostomy.
- Any attempt to re-insert a tracheostomy should be quickly abandoned if unsuccessful.
    - A well-formed track from skin to the tracheal stoma takes >72 hours to form following surgical tracheostomy or >7 days after percutaneous tracheostomy.
- If unable to ventilate through the stoma, re-establish the airway in the usual fashion. Tilt the head back to extend the head on the neck, perform a jaw thrust. If necessary insert an oral airway (Guedel).
- Note that if 'bag and mask' ventilation is attempted, air will escape through the stoma. In this situation, get a colleague to occlude the stoma by applying pressure over it with gauze swabs or a pad.
- Tracheal intubation may be needed. It may be necessary to push the tracheal tube distal to the stoma. (Use an 'uncut' tube.)
- If the patient is breathing adequately at this point, there may be no need to artificially assist ventilation. Check the oxygen saturation with a pulse oximeter and administer oxygen as required via a facemask or resuscitation bag with an oxygen reservoir.
- If artificial ventilation is needed, use a resuscitation bag and mask in the standard fashion.
- Maintain occlusion of the stoma as described earlier to prevent an air leak. Capnography will confirm tracheal intubation. Measurement of oxygen saturation with a pulse oximeter will confirm adequacy of oxygenation.

- At this point the patient is safe, with a patent airway and adequate respiration. Do not panic.
- A decision about re-insertion of the tracheostomy tube can now be made by the senior anaesthetist.

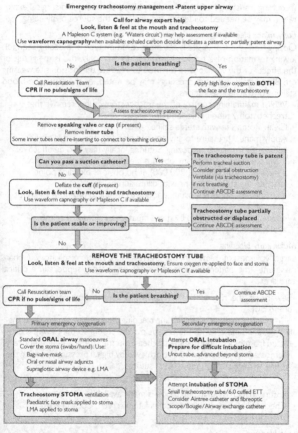

Figure 25.1 Emergency tracheostomy management—patent upper airway. Reproduced from McGrath BA, Bates L, Atkinson D, Moore JA. Multidisciplinary guidelines for the management of tracheostomy and laryngectomy airway emergencies. *Anaesthesia.* 2012 Jun 26. doi: 10.1111/j.1365-2044.2012.07217, with permission from the Association of Anaesthetists of Great Britain & Ireland/Blackwell Publishing Ltd.

Bleeding from a tracheostomy

Bleeding is the most common complication of tracheostomy.
- Bleeding may occur early (within 48 hours of formation of the tracheostomy).
- Bleeding may be late (several days afterwards).

It may be minor (settles with simple conservative management) or major (requiring transfusion of blood and/or blood products) and surgical exploration may be needed to identify and deal with the source of bleeding.

Early minor bleeding

Oozing from the stoma site is the most common type of bleeding seen following formation of a tracheostomy. Most commonly, this is the result of the effects of the vasoconstrictor used to infiltrate the incision site wearing off. Blood staining of the dressings may be noted, or there may be blood staining of tracheal secretions.
- Whilst maintaining control of the tracheostomy tube, remove the tracheostomy tube holder and dressing.
- Clean stoma site with sterile saline.
- Apply manual pressure to any obvious bleeding point—this may be sufficient to stop minor oozing. Suturing locally may also be effective.
- If still bleeding, infiltrate any obvious bleeding point with dilute adrenaline (1:80,000 to 1:200,000). If no obvious bleeding point, infiltrate the stoma margins with dilute adrenaline.
- If still oozing, apply Kaltostat® packing to stoma to promote local clot formation.
- If bleeding is not stopped by these measures, refer for surgical exploration.

Major early bleeding

Large volumes of blood in the trachea may cause respiratory embarrassment—the patient may need further respiratory support in a critical care area.

Beware of the risk of the tracheostomy tube becoming occluded by blood clot.

In most situations of significant bleeding, secure the airway by translaryngeal intubation with the cuff below the stoma so the airway is protected from blood entering the trachea from the stoma. Then temporary haemostasis of the stoma can be achieved by digital pressure, packing the wound with gauze or deep tension sutures.

- Ensure that cross-matched blood is made available.
- Check full blood count and a coagulation screen. Correct any abnormalities in the standard way.

Late bleeding

Late bleeding may occur because of erosion of blood vessels in and around the stoma site. This is more likely if there has been infection of the stoma site. Such bleeding may settle with conservative management, as described in the early bleed guideline.

Late bleeding may be the result of erosion of a major artery in the root of the neck where there has been pressure from the tracheostomy tube itself or the cuff.

- *Don't panic.*
- Call for help—senior medical and nursing staff, other AHPs with tracheostomy care skills.
- Reassure the patient.
- Bleeding may be temporarily reduced or stopped by applying finger pressure to the root of the neck in the sternal notch, or by inflating the tracheostomy tube cuff (if present) with a 50mL syringe of air. This inflation should be done slowly and steadily to inflate the balloon to a maximum volume without bursting it. This may be anywhere between 10mL and 35mL.
- Urgent referral for surgical exploration must be made.
- Ensure that cross-matched blood is made available.
- Check full blood count and a coagulation screen. Correct any abnormalities in the standard way.

Weaning and decannulation

Once on low-level respiratory support, the time spent breathing through a T piece is gradually increased. The cuff is normally deflated at this stage, allowing use of a speaking valve. Use of decannulation cap is not required, and will increase work of breathing unnecessarily. When the patient has not required respiratory support for an acceptable period (at least 24 hours) decannulation may be undertaken if there is:

- Patent upper airway
- Adequate cough for amount of secretions
- Intact bulbar function.

Use of a minitracheostomy has been shown to reduce sputum retention and the need for re-intubation in thoracic surgical patients.

Further reading

Bonde P, Papachristos I, McCraith A, Kelly B, Wilson C, McGuigan JA, *et al*. Sputum retention after lung operation: Prospective, randomized trial shows superiority of prophylactic minitracheostomy in high-risk patients. *Ann Thoracic Surg* 2002;74(1)196–203.

Intensive Care Society. *Standards for the Care of Adult Patients with a Temporary Tracheostomy.* 2008. ⅃ <http://www.ics.ac.uk/ics-homepage/guidelines-standards/>.

Terragni PP, Antonelli M, Fumagalli R, Faggiano C, Berardino M, Pallavicini FB, *et al*. Early vs late tracheotomy for prevention of pneumonia in mechanically ventilated adult ICU patients: a randomized controlled trial. *JAMA* 2010;303(15):1483–9.

Extubation

Removal of the ETT (extubation) is undertaken after successful weaning from mechanical ventilation. In patients with COPD or neuromuscular disease extubation may precede fully completed weaning.

Pre-conditions for extubation

- Adequate oxygenation (PaO_2:FiO_2 ratio >27kPa).
- Normal $PaCO_2$ (except in those known to be chronically hypercapnic)
- Adequate level of consciousness, compatible with maintaining an airway and clearing secretions (obeying commands)
- Adequate cough (to deal with current secretion volume)
- Adequate bulbar function
- Adequate respiratory muscle strength (vital capacity 12–15mL/kg)
- Adequate cuff leak in patients ventilated for >24 hours (see 'Cuff leak test' later in this topic)
- Successful trial of spontaneous breathing (see ☐ Weaning strategies, p. 283).

Process of extubation

Preparation

- Drugs and equipment for reintubation should be immediately available including equipment for a difficult airway.
- Prepare an oxygen mask and system capable of delivering humidified oxygen.

Process

- Often a two-person job.
- Inform the patient and surrounding staff.
- Ensure enteral feed is stopped (preferably for 4 hours).
- Aspirate gastric contents via NG tube.
- Sit patient up.
- Suction mouth and oropharynx and aspirate subglottic drain if applicable.
- Undo tube ties.
- In order to deal with secretions present above cuff, deflate the pilot balloon of the ETT while suction catheter remains in trachea.
- Withdraw the ETT with constant aspiration of the suction catheter.
- Administer humidified oxygen.

Extubation failure

Post extubation failure and re-intubation is associated with a marked increase in mortality and ICU length of stay. Signs include stridor, dyspnoea, sweating, use of accessory muscles, tachypnoea, tachycardia, hypotension or hypertension, hypoxaemia, and hypercapnia.

Ideally, identify the cause of extubation failure before reintubation—it is often difficult in retrospect. Perform an examination, arrange for ECG and echocardiogram, CXR, and SvO_2. If stridor is present, fibreoptic laryngoscopy will delineate the underlying aetiology. Often the degree of respiratory distress will appropriately curtail these investigations.

Causes of extubation failure

Early failure is usually due to upper airway swelling, LV failure, or inadequate assessment.

Stridor

Post-extubation stridor can be caused by laryngospasm, laryngeal oedema, or excessive dynamic airway collapse and tracheobronchomalacia. It is often under-recognized and occurs in 10–15% of patients who are extubated after >24 hours of ventilation. Risk factors include medical admissions, female sex, traumatic or difficult intubations, cuff pressure >30cmH$_2$O, prolonged intubation, and a history of self extubation.

Cuff leak test

- During IPPV a leak of <110mL or <18% tidal volume predicts post extubation stridor.
- If breathing spontaneously, the presence of an audible leak while using PEEP 10cmH$_2$O is a sensible alternative measure.
- Steroids reduce post-extubation stridor in those with inadequate cuff leak (dexamethasone 4mg four times a day for 24–48 hours).

Management

Laryngospasm, excessive dynamic airway collapse or tracheobronchomalacia:
- Application of high-flow oxygen
- CPAP
- Reintubation if these measures fail.

Laryngeal oedema:
- Nebulized adrenaline (the levo-isomer is recommended, though with poor supporting evidence).
- Dexamethasone 4mg four times daily.
- In the presence of significant respiratory distress re: intubation should not be delayed.

Left ventricular failure

Extubation places considerable strain on the left ventricle.
- Removal of positive intrathoracic pressure increases preload and afterload
- Extubation can be frightening—↑ sympathetic drive may add to myocardial work.
- ↑ minute ventilation will increase oxygen demand.

Underlying causes should be treated, full medical therapy should be instituted, and aggressive diuresis carried out before further attempt at extubation, even if LV function improves post reintubation.

Respiratory dysfunction

Respiratory dysfunction post extubation is often multifactorial:
- Loss of positive intrathoracic pressure and alveolar hypoventilation due to muscle weakness cause atelectasis. The result is ↑ work of breathing and poor gas exchange.
- Large volume or viscous secretions cause alveolar hypoventilation, consolidation, ↑ work of breathing, and poor gas exchange.

- A poor cough or associated muscle weakness may exacerbate both these problems.
- Wheeze (asthma, COPD, LV failure).
- LV dysfunction.

Inadequate assessment

Patients whose underlying pathology has not resolved sufficiently, or who have not met the preconditions for extubation (described earlier) are unlikely to tolerate extubation.

Non-invasive ventilation

- Use of NIV to manage respiratory failure post extubation has been shown to increase mortality. These patients should be reintubated.
- Use of NIV electively in hypercapnic patients or patients with COPD reduces the rate of reintubation.

Reintubation

- Reintubation may be complicated by laryngeal oedema following prolonged intubation.
- Avoid suxamethonium in patients at risk of critical illness polymyoneuropathy (severe sepsis or prolonged mechanical ventilation). Severe hyperkalaemia may result.

Respiratory management

Positive pressure ventilation

Modes of mechanical ventilation

Positive pressure ventilators
Ventilators and ventilator modes may be classified according to input power, mode of triggering, inspiratory characteristics, mode of cycling, the pattern of mandatory and spontaneous breaths, and method of synchronization.

Input power
Input is either electrical or pneumatic.

Triggering—the start of inspiration
Ventilators measure pressure, volume, flow, and time. Inspiration is started (triggered) when one of these variables reaches a preset value. Breaths may be triggered by the patient or ventilator. If the respiratory rate is set at 10/min, a controlled mechanical breath will be commenced every 6 seconds (time triggering). For patient-triggered breaths, it is usually a change in flow or pressure which results in the start of a supported spontaneous breath (e.g. pressure support ventilation, PSV) or a mandatory breath (e.g. synchronized intermittent mandatory ventilation (SIMV) in the synchronization window, or assist control ventilation (ACV)). Alternate triggers are possible (e.g. diaphragmatic contraction or chest wall motion in children).

Inspiratory phase
Control mode
Ventilators are either pressure controllers, or flow (or volume) controllers. In practice flow and volume controllers behave almost identically (direct control of flow means indirect control of volume and vice versa) and both are called 'volume controlled ventilation' (VCV). Most VCV uses flow control.

Pressure control ventilation versus volume control ventilation
The diagrams demonstrate the difference between a pressure-controlled and a volume-controlled breath.

With pressure control, inspiratory pressure is chosen by the clinician (1a). Flow in a passive patient is decelerating (1b first curve). With increasing patient effort sine wave flow becomes more prominent. Airway pressure is controlled, but the volume delivered depends on respiratory system impedance and inspiratory time (1c).

Usually with volume control, TV and inspiratory flow are chosen by the clinician (inspiratory flow is often set indirectly by choosing the respiratory rate, inspiratory:expiratory ratio, and tidal volume, e.g. RR 20, I:E 1:2, TV 600mL=1 second for inspiration, therefore inspiratory flow of 36L/min; 2b). Delivered volume is controlled, but airway pressure is dependent on resistance (for peak pressure) and compliance (for plateau pressure) (2a).

No benefit in significant outcomes has ever been demonstrated for either mode over the other. Many of the trials of ventilatory strategies use volume control ventilation. Compared with VCV, PCV has the following theoretical advantages:

- Alveolar pressure is limited and cannot be higher than the set inspiratory pressure.
- Peak airway pressures will be lower for an equivalent tidal volume.
- For a given peak airway pressure, mean airway pressure is higher. Oxygenation may therefore be improved (but will also depend on the plateau pressure and PEEP).
- There may be improved distribution of ventilation. There is less end inspiratory gradient of pressure among regional units with heterogeneous time constants. CO_2 elimination is improved.

The main disadvantage of PCV is the variation in tidal volume. In addition, when there is vigorous patient inspiratory effort, pleural pressure drops significantly and the transpulmonary pressure (one of the crucial causes of ventilator-induced lung injury (VILI)) may be high.

Studies do not demonstrate a difference in the incidence of VILI and there are similar haemodynamic consequences.

Modern ventilators can deliver breaths with characteristics of both types of breath, called dual control or hybrid breaths (e.g. pressure regulated volume control, where pressure control and decelerating flow patterns are combined with volume cycling).

Limit

The term limit refers to any variable which reaches a preset value before inspiration ends. It sustains inspiration. 'Limit' is sometimes interchangeable with 'control', e.g. pressure-controlled breaths are equivalent to pressure-limited breaths which are equivalent to pressure-targeted breaths. This terminology may also lead to confusion: the phrase 'volume limited' usually means flow limited and volume cycled (VCV).

Inspiratory to expiratory cycling—the start of expiration

Expiration starts when a preset value of flow, time, volume (or pressure) is reached. Mandatory breaths are generally time cycled (PCV) or volume cycled (VCV). Spontaneous supported breaths (PSV) are usually flow cycled (expiration usually starts at 25–33% of peak inspiratory flow. This is adjustable on some ventilators).

Pressure cycling is now only used as a safety backup for other forms of cycling, i.e. it will terminate the breath if pressure rises to the preset limit.

Mandatory vs spontaneous and patient-ventilator synchrony

Mandatory breaths are machine triggered or cycled. Mandatory breaths that are patient triggered are called assisted.

Spontaneous breaths are patient triggered and cycled. Spontaneous breaths may be supported or unsupported.

Synchrony is the agreement between the patient's own (neural) and the ventilator (mechanical) inspiratory and expiratory time, and includes the matching of patient effort with delivered tidal volume (more effort should result in ↑ volume). Each mode of ventilation has specific rules governing interaction with the patient. These rules are made clear in all ventilator manuals, but this subject is outside the scope of this chapter. As an example we will examine the differences between pressure SIMV (P-SIMV) and BIPAP:

P-SIMV and BIPAP are identical in a passive patient.

In an active patient, patient ventilator interaction during expiration is the same. There are two expiratory time windows. During the first period of expiration, the patient is allowed to breathe spontaneously or with support (PSV). During the second (trigger) window, patient effort will trigger a time-cycled mandatory breath.

The modes, however, differ during inspiration. With BIPAP, the patient can breathe throughout inspiration (with a floating valve opening to prevent excessive airway pressure). Patient efforts are allowed, and superimposed on the time-cycled inspiratory pressure. Cycling to expiration is also synchronized with patient expiration. With P-SIMV, patient effort is unrecognized during inspiration, and may result in breath termination due to a breach of the high pressure safety limit.

Synchrony

It is important to recognize that no current mode of ventilation that uses pneumatic signals to trigger and cycle (including modes such as PSV/ assisted spontaneous breathing) is without significant synchrony problems. Difficulties include inspiratory trigger delay, ineffective triggering, double triggering, auto triggering, inspiratory time extension, early expiratory cycling, and failure of expiratory cycling. Neurally adjusted ventilatory assist (NAVA) may reduce some of the common difficulties by using diaphragmatic contraction to trigger breaths and to guide support levels.

Complications encountered in mechanical ventilation

Complications of endotracheal tube
- Ventilator-associated pneumonia
- Tracheal stenosis
- Vocal cord injury
- Tracheo-oesophageal fistula
- Sinusitis.

Complications of mechanical ventilation
- VILI
- Air leaks including bronchopleural fistulae
- Oxygen toxicity
- Reduction in CO
- Reduction in renal or splanchnic blood supply
- Fluid retention (↑ renin, angiotensin, aldosterone, and antidiuretic hormone; ↓ atrial natriuretic peptide)
- Ventilator-induced diaphragmatic dysfunction.

Complications due to immobility
- VTE
- Pressure sores.

Complications related to critical illness
- GI bleeding, GI dysmotility, endocrine disease, polymyoneuropathy.

Effects of positive intrathoracic pressure

The mean intrathroracic pressure depends on the PEEP, plateau pressure, and time spent in inspiration (the I:E ratio).

Cardiovascular side effects due to heart–lung interactions are common. Both changes in lung volume and changes in intrathoracic pressure contribute to these consequences. Full discussion is beyond the scope of this chapter.

Respiratory side effects constitute the best documented short- and long-term causes of morbidity and mortality related to ventilation. These range from sudden onset of tension pneumothorax to the development of diffuse alveolar damage, the release of inflammatory mediators, and subsequent other organ dysfunction (VILI).

Potential benefits of positive intrathoracic pressure
- Alveolar recruitment:
  - Reduced shunt
  - ↑ V/Q.
  - Improved compliance and reduced work of breathing.
- Reduced LV preload and afterload in cardiogenic pulmonary oedema.
- Reduced PVR by increasing lung volumes towards normal and reversing hypoxic pulmonary vasoconstriction.

Potential harms
- ↑ shunt fraction—elevating mean airway pressure will increase PVR in compliant, healthy areas of lung and divert blood to consolidated areas.
- ↑ deadspace—↓ blood flow to ventilated areas, especially in apical regions.
- ↓ compliance—overdistended lung on the flat upper portion of the P/V (compliance) curve.
- ↑ PVR (if lung is overdistended).
- ↓ CO:
  - Reduced LV preload or↑ PVR in normo- or hypovolaemic states.
  - Reduced CO may increase V/Q, but will reduce oxygen delivery and SvO_2.

Detrimental heart lung interactions can be minimized by preventing both hyperinflation and alveolar derecruitment, reducing work of breathing, preventing volume overload during weaning, and avoiding negative pressure swings in intrathoracic pressure during spontaneous breathing.

Expiration

Expiration is passive in all modes except high frequency oscillation. PEEP is almost always applied in critically unwell patients. It increases FRC, recruits alveoli, reduces shunt, helps prevent atelectrauma and reduces preload and afterload. A full discussion of the best way to set the level of PEEP is out with the scope of this chapter.

Ventilator Induced Lung Injury

This term encompasses barotrauma (injury due to excessive pressure) and volutrauma (injury due to excessive volume) – in combination these produce alveolar strain (defined as the ratio between the amount of gas volume delivered compared with the amount of aerated lung receiving it). Crucially, damage is also caused by atelectrauma (injury due to repeated opening and closing of alveoli) and biotrauma (distal organ dysfunction caused by release of inflammatory mediators because of VILI). Preventing VILI is difficult and the best way to do so is not established. In ARDS, avoid plateau pressures > 30cm H2O, use tidal volumes of no more than 6ml/kg of ideal body weight, select PEEP to prevent end expiratory alveolar closure without increasing alveolar strain (see further reading), and perhaps use intermittent recruitment manoeuvres. These techniques, in combination with permissive hypercapnia and permissive hypoxia, are together termed 'Lung Protective Ventilation'.

In concept, High Frequency Oscillatory Ventilation seemed the ideal way to achieve these ends, but two recent trials have suggested that at best outcomes are not improved, or that mortality may be worse when using this technique on unselected patients with ARDS.

Acknowledgement

This section is adapted from *Anaesthesia & Intensive Care Medicine*, 14, 10, Martin Hughes et al., 'Ventilatory support in the intensive care unit', pp. 466–471, Copyright 2013, with permission from Elsevier.

Further reading

Ferguson N.D. et al. High Frequency Oscillation in Early Acute Respiratory Distress Syndrome. *N Engl J Med* 2013;368:795–805.

Hughes M, Black R (eds). *Advanced Respiratory Critical Care*. Oxford: Oxford University Press; 2011.

Pinsky MR. Heart lung interactions. *Curr Opin Crit Care* 2007;13(5):528–31.

Strachan L, Hughes M. Ventilatory support in the intensive care unit. *Anaesthes Intens Care Med* 2010;11(11):469–473.

.Young D. et al. High frequency oscillation for acute Respiratory Distress Syndrome. *N Engl J Med* 2013;368:806–13.

CPAP and non-invasive ventilation

CPAP

CPAP is the application of constant positive airway pressure throughout the respiratory cycle in the spontaneously breathing patient. CPAP mainly improves oxygenation (see 📖 Effects of positive intrathoracic pressure p. 279). Effect on work of breathing is variable and depends on respiratory mechanics.

NIV

NIV usually refers to the application of higher inspiratory (inspiratory positive airway pressure (IPAP)) than expiratory positive airway pressure (EPAP). It is usually patient triggered and flow cycled. It will improve oxygenation, increase minute ventilation, and usually reduce work of breathing.

Contraindications to CPAP and NIV
- Respiratory arrest
- Unprotected airway/reduced conscious level
- Upper airway obstruction
- Inability to clear secretions
- Haemodynamic instability
- Untreated pneumothorax
- Base of skull or facial fractures.

Complications of NIV
- Patient discomfort
- Pressure sores
- Gastric insufflation
- Aspiration
- Barotrauma.

Use of CPAP and NIV

Non-invasive ventilation modes are useful in the treatment of reversible disease processes of limited duration. It has limited application in the treatment of prolonged disease processes like ALI.

Cardiogenic pulmonary oedema
↑ lung water secondary to interstitial and alveolar oedema increases the elastic workload of the lung and reduces compliance. CPAP recruits alveoli, reduces intrapulmonary shunt, and reduces preload and afterload. It often results in a rapid improvement in the patient's condition, and reduces mortality. The addition of an IPAP does not improve outcome.

Acute respiratory failure in COPD
In COPD, EPAP overcomes the ↑ threshold load due to intrinsic PEEP, and IPAP compensates for the additional inspiratory resistance from bronchoconstriction. Work of breathing is reduced and tidal volumes are increased.

In hypercapnic, acidotic exacerbations of COPD, BIPAP reduces intubation rates, and reduces in-hospital mortality. The risk reduction is directly proportional to the severity of the respiratory acidosis.

Others

Evidence for the use of NIV in other disease processes is limited. If the patient requires respiratory support continuously (as opposed to COPD where breaks can be taken), or for a long period (as opposed to LV failure where improvement is often relatively rapid), a tight-fitting facemask is often eventually poorly tolerated because of facial discomfort or skin breakdown.

In addition, gastric insufflation, difficulty clearing secretions, and an absence of airway protection reduce the effectiveness of prolonged use of CPAP and NIV. Where no clinical improvement is seen, intubation should be considered.

Used prophylactically after extubation it reduces reintubation in patients with COPD or who are hypercapnic pre extubation. It does not work well for respiratory failure post extubation.

Further reading

Burns KEA, Adhikari NKJ, Keenan SP, Meade M. Use of non-invasive ventilation to wean critically ill adults off invasive ventilation: meta-analysis and systematic review. *BMJ* 2009;338:b1574.

Gray A, Goodacre S, Newby DE, Masson M, Sampson F, Nicholl J; on behalf of the 3 CPO trialists. Noninvasive ventilation in acute cardiogenic pulmonary oedema. *NEJM* 2008;359(2):142–51.

Peter JV, Moran JL. Noninvasive ventilation in exacerbations of chronic obstructive pulmonary disease: implications of different meta-analytic strategies. *Ann Intern Med* 2004;141(5):W78–9.

Peter JV, Moran JL, Phillips-Hughes J, Graham P, Bersten AD. Effect of non-invasive positive pressure ventilation (NIPPV) on mortality in patients with acute cardiogenic pulmonary oedema: a meta-analysis. *Lancet* 2006;367:115–63.

Ram FSF, Picot J, Lightowler J, Wedzicha JA. Non-invasive positive pressure ventilation for treatment of respiratory failure due to exacerbations of chronic obstructive pulmonary disease. *Cochrane Database Syst Rev* 2004;3:CD004104.

Weng C, Zhao T, Liu Q, Fu CJ, Sun F, Ma YL, *et al.* Meta-analysis: non-invasive ventilation in acute cardiogenic pulmonary edema. *Ann Intern Med* 2010;152(9):590–600.

Weaning strategies

Weaning is the process of liberation from mechanical ventilation. It need not be a prolonged process, and many patients are weaned immediately postoperatively. This chapter deals with weaning from mechanical ventilation in the presence of acute or chronic respiratory disease.

Unnecessary prolongation of ventilation is costly and associated with an ↑ risk of ventilator-associated pneumonia, lung injury, and delirium. Risk factors for prolonged weaning include old age, severity of acute illness, duration of mechanical ventilation, chronic respiratory disease, and neuromuscular or musculoskeletal disorders.

Titration of respiratory support

A process of active weaning is different from the titration of respiratory support while the wean screen (see later in topic) excludes the patient from a spontaneous breathing trial. This is the routine management of ventilatory support, progressing from high FiO_2 and airway pressures towards a spontaneous breathing trial.

Consider both the support required for oxygenation, and the support required for work of breathing. In general, FiO_2 is reduced to ≤0.6 before there is a significant reduction in mean airway pressure. At this point, PEEP is lowered if oxygenation is acceptable. Inspiratory pressures, on the other hand, are reduced as tidal volume improves with ↑ compliance, and if work of breathing is reasonable.

Assessment of suitability for weaning

Prediction of successful weaning has been the subject of much investigation. Minute ventilation, maximal inspiratory pressure, $P_{0.1}$/Pimax and CROP score (Compliance Respiratory rate Oxygenation and Pressure) are all associated with an ↑ chance of success. Unfortunately, the likelihood ratios are not large enough to make these measurements a real alternative to spontaneous breathing trials.

As well as a daily sedation vacation, a wean screen should be completed. If the wean screen is passed, a spontaneous breathing trial is undertaken and suitability for extubation (see 📖 Extubation, p. 272) considered.

Wean screen
- Adequate resolution of underlying disease
- PaO_2/FiO_2 > 25kPa, PEEP ≤8cmH_2O
- Low-dose inotropic or vasoconstrictor support
- Capable of spontaneous breaths.

Spontaneous breathing trials
Spontaneous breathing trials do not take account of the preconditions to extubation (see 📖 Extubation, p. 272). However, they are currently the best predictor of a patient's ability to breathe independently.

A spontaneous breathing trial is 30–120 minutes long in uncomplicated patients. After a prolonged weaning process, progressively increasing the duration of the trial until the trial lasts ≥24 hours may be appropriate. Traditionally, spontaneous breathing was assessed using a T-piece. Many clinicians add PEEP of 5 to reproduce physiological PEEP, and pressure support of 5–8cmH_2O to overcome the resistance of the tube. Too much support will lead to an ↑ failed extubation rate. Too little support will lead to unnecessary failure of the spontaneous breathing trial and delayed extubation.

The purpose of the trial is to reproduce the postextubation work of breathing conditions before extubation. While in most patients PS and PEEP will most accurately replicate these conditions, there are two subgroups in whom a T-piece trial may be useful:

• Patients with known LV systolic dysfunction. Assessment without the beneficial effects of PEEP is helpful.
• Patients with known or potential upper airway swelling (e.g. prolonged intubation, significant oedema) where the postextubation work of breathing is likely to be higher.

As the majority of patients in the CICU setting have an element of LV systolic dysfunction, a successful T-piece trial will reduce the rate of failed extubation.

A spontaneous breathing trial should be discontinued if there is:

• Respiratory compromise: PaO_2/FiO_2 <25kPa, respiratory rate >35 breaths/minute or increase of >50%, accessory muscle use, fatigue
• Cardiovascular instability: systolic BP >180mmHg or <90mmHg, HR >120bpm.
• Neurological dysfunction: agitation, anxiety, sweating, or reduction in GCS score.

The daily sedation hold, wean screen, and spontaneous breathing trial constitute a weaning protocol. Despite a reluctance to use such protocols, in trials they outperform or match more traditional methods of weaning.

Management of weaning failure

Identify factors which increase respiratory load or decrease respiratory capacity.

Respiratory

CT chest is increasingly the investigation of choice in ICU. It allows accurate assessment of lung parenchyma and pleural disease:

• Exclude infection. If in doubt perform bronchoalveolar lavage.
• Drain pleural effusions, unless small bilateral transudates and diuresis is underway.
• Treat bronchospasm.
• Reduce FiO_2 to achieve a normal SpO_2 for that patient.
• Normalize $PaCO_2$ unless chronically hypercapnic. If respiratory acidosis has resulted in compensatory metabolic alkalosis, several days of mandatory mode of ventilation (with high MV), combined with acetazolamide (to eliminate more quickly the metabolic alkalosis) is reasonable. Continue until bicarbonate is normal.
• Bronchoscopy may help to re-expand lobar or segmental collapse.

Cardiovascular

• If echocardiography is normal, repeat during a spontaneous breathing trial.
• Treat LV dysfunction, myocardial ischaemia and dysrhythmias.
• Aggressive diuresis—clear the CXR.

Central nervous system
- Avoid oversedation.
- Reduce precipitating factors for delirium including benzodiazepines.

Metabolic
- Correct hypophosphataemia.
- Optimize nutrition.

General management
- Draw up an individual plan and keep it at the bedside. Deviation from the plan should be clinically justified.
- During the day, progressively wean pressure support and increase the time with no respiratory support.
- During a prolonged wean, night time should be a period of rest to allow sleep, re-recruit the lung, and correct hypercapnia. PSV alone is associated with ↑ sleep disturbance (compared with assist control ventilation) because of apnoeas and micro-arousals: a mandatory backup rate prevents this.
- Demedicalize the environment: TV, reading materials, and items from home including normal clothes.
- Sitting improves functional residual capacity, and promotes normality.
- Encourage eating and drinking.
- Speaking valves improve morale and vocal cord function.

Remember the possibility of long-term (home) ventilation for some patients who are unable to wean.

Circulatory support

Pharmacological support

There is a lack of robust clinical evidence demonstrating a positive impact on survival concerning the use of vasoactive agents. Their use is considered part of supportive care allowing time for definitive treatment of underlying disease processes. This treatment might involve antibiotics for sepsis, management of arrhythmias, or, in the context of cardiothoracic critical care, interventions such as PCI, surgical revascularization, or the institution of mechanical support (discussed in Mechanical circulatory support, p. 294).

The selection and safe use of a particular vasoactive agent is based on knowledge of its cardiovascular effects, clinical indications, and an understanding of its clinical use.

Inotropic agents

Catecholamines

Catecholamines exert their cardiovascular effects via activity at specific adrenergic (a_1, β_1, β_2) and dopaminergic (D_1) receptors. Sensitive β receptor effects are evident at low plasma concentrations while α effects become more prominent at higher concentrations.

Myocardial contractility is enhanced by activity at β_1 receptors leading to ↑ levels of cAMP and intracellular Ca^{2+} with the inevitable consequence of ↑ myocardial oxygen consumption (MVO_2).

Dobutamine

- Synthetic catecholamine.
- Direct β_1 >β_2 agonist (3:1 ratio) with some α_1 activity.

Dose-dependent CVS effects:
- ↑ contractility (β_1 with α_1).
- ↑ HR and AV conduction (β_1).
- Vasodilatation (β_2 with mixed α_1 agonism/antagonism) at low doses (<5mcg/kg/min).
- Variable effects on vasculature at intermediate doses.
- Vasoconstriction (α_1) at higher doses (>15mcg/kg/min).

Predominant effects are increases in SV and CO with SVR moderately reduced or unchanged. MAP may thus fall, remain unchanged, or rise with increasing CO. ↑ MVO_2 is attenuated by a reduction in preload/afterload and offset by augmented myocardial blood flow.

Clinical indications:
- First-line agent to support borderline CO post cardiac surgery.
- Low CO (DHF, cardiogenic shock, sepsis-induced myocardial dysfunction).

Clinical use:
- Dosing: 2.5–25mcg/kg/min; max. 40mcg/kg/min.
- Onset 2 minutes; peak effect 10 minutes; plasma half-life 2 minutes.
- Addition of a vasopressor (e.g. noradrenaline) is often required to maintain MAP.
- Increases HR more than adrenaline for similar increases in CO and may be used as indirect chronotrope.
- Tachycardia and arrhythmias limit upper dose.
- Tachyphylaxis occurs after 48–72 hours.

Dopamine
- Endogenous catecholamine precursor to noradrenaline.
- α_1, β_1/β_2, D_1 agonist with release of neuronal noradrenaline.

Dose-dependent CVS effects:
- ↑ contractility (β_1)
- ↑ HR and AV conduction (β_1)
- Vasodilatation at lower doses (0.5–3mcg/kg/min)Renal, mesenteric, coronary (D_1), peripheral vessels (β_2)
- Mild vasoconstriction (α_1) (3–10mcg/kg/min)
- Vasoconstriction (α_1) at higher doses (10–20mcg/kg/min)

Predominant effects are an increase in SV and CO with mild increases in SVR and ↑ MAP. Vasoconstriction at higher doses raises SVR and MAP but also increases PVR and MVO_2.

Renal effects:
- ↑ renal blood flow via ↑ CO (β_1) and vasodilatation (D_1).
- ↑ urine output secondary to ↑ renal blood flow and enhanced natriuesis (D_1) without altering creatinine clearance

Clinical indications:
- First-line agent to support borderline CO post cardiac surgery.
- Shock (cardiogenic, vasodilatory).
- Augmentation of diuresis in DHF.

Clinical use:
- Dosing: 2–20mcg/kg/min; max. 50mcg/kg/min.
- Peak effect 5–10 minutes; plasma half-life 2 minutes.
- Plasma concentrations unpredictable due to variable clearance in the critically ill.
- Tachyarrhythmias may limit use even at lower doses.
- If inadequate response at <10mcg/kg/min consider switch to adrenaline or addition of a second agent.
- Low-dose dopamine is not effective in the prevention or treatment of acute renal failure.

Adrenaline
- Endogenous catecholamine.
- Potent α_1, β_1/β_2 agonist.

Dose-dependent CVS effects:
- ↑ contractility (β_1, β_2, α_1).
- ↑ HR and AV conduction (β_1).
- Vasodilatation (β_2) at low doses (<0.03mcg/kg/min).
- Vasoconstriction (α_1) at higher doses (>0.03mcg/kg/min).

Increases in SV, HR, CO, and SVR result in significant increases in MAP and MVO_2. In septic shock, increases in MAP are achieved predominantly by increasing SV.

Additional effects:
- Bronchodilation (β_2).
- Mast cell stabilization.

- ↑ lactate levels (enhanced glycogenolysis and glycolysis with reduced pyruvate utilization).
- ↑ glucose levels (enhanced glycogenolysis).

Clinical indications:
- First-line agent to support low CO post cardiac surgery.
- Shock (cardiogenic, vasodilatory).
- Bronchospasm/anaphylaxis.
- Cardiac arrest.

Clinical use:
- Dosing: 0.01–0.5mcg/kg/min; >0.05mcg/kg/min rarely indicated following cardiac surgery.
- Greater efficacy than the other catecholamines.
- Can be used in combination with a phosphodiesterase (PDE) inhibitor to augment CO without the same increases in afterload and MVO_2.
- Tachyarrhythmias remain relatively common.

Phosphodiesterase inhibitors
Milrinone and enoximone
- Inhibit PDE breakdown of cAMP in cardiac myocytes and vascular smooth muscle.

Dose-dependent CVS effects:
- ↑ contractility.
- Enhanced diastolic relaxation.
- Modest increase HR and AV conduction.
- Vasodilatation.

Increases in SV and CO are achieved via moderate increases in contractility along with reduced SVR/PVR. MAP is commonly reduced. Reductions in preload/afterload have a beneficial effect on MVO_2.

Clinical indications:
- Second-line agents to support low CO post cardiac surgery.
- Low CO with raised SVR.
- Biventricular or RV failure associated with ↑ PVR, e.g. before and after cardiac transplant, mitral valve surgery.

Clinical use:
- Milrinone: loading dose 25–50mcg/kg; infusion 0.375–0.75mcg/kg/min; Half-life 2–4 hours.
- Enoximone: loading dose 0.5–1mg/kg; infusion 2.5–20mcg/kg/min; half-life 4–6 hours.
- Long half-life means titration to effect is achieved over hours rather than minutes and effects (beneficial and adverse) are similarly prolonged.
- Synergistic effect on CO when used with catecholamines.
- Vasodilatation, which limits clinical use, often requires the addition of a vasopressor (e.g. noradrenaline).
- Useful in the setting of adrenergic receptor downregulation, e.g. chronic HF, or after chronic β-agonist administration.
- Less tachycardia and risk of arrhythmias than with dobutamine.

Levosimendan

In common with other members of the calcium sensitizer class levosimendan exerts its main inotropic effects by increasing calcium binding to troponin C. It also opens ATP sensitive K^+ channels and inhibits PDE.

Dose-dependent CVS effects

- ↑ contractility (Ca^{2+} sensitization).
- Vasodilatation (K^+ channel opening).
- Enhanced diastolic relaxation (PDE inhibitor activity).

Overall effects are similar to those of PDE inhibitors with increases in SV and CO and a reduction in SVR/PVR. MAP is reduced or unchanged. Minimal effect on MVO_2 while coronary blood flow is ↑.

Clinical indications

- Currently third-line agent to support CO post cardiac surgery.
- Low CO (cardiogenic shock, DHF).

Clinical use

- Loading dose 6–12mcg/kg; infusion 0.05–0.2mcg/kg/min for 24 hours.
- Active metabolites; effects persist for up to 9 days.
- May also be useful in adrenergic receptor downregulation.
- When compared with dobutamine it provides similar improvements in CO with smaller increases in MVO_2.
- Some evidence to suggest improved outcomes in cardiac surgery.
- No long-term survival benefit over dobutamine in treatment of acute DHF.
- Potential for QT prolongation and ventricular arrhythmias.

Vasopressors

Noradrenaline

- Endogenous catecholamine.
- Potent α_1 agonist; modest β_1 and limited β_2 activity.

Dose-dependent CVS effects

- Vasoconstriction (α_1) characterizes its clinical effect.
- Modest increases in contractility (β_1).
- Minimal increase in HR (β_1), or reflex decrease (α_1).
- Increases PVR.

Increases in SVR, with modest increases in SV result in elevated systolic, diastolic and pulse pressure with minimal impact on CO. ↑ afterload and contractility result in ↑ MVO_2 though coronary flow is ↑ secondary to elevated diastolic BP.

Clinical indications

- Shock (vasodilatory).

Clinical use

- Dosing: 0.01–0.3mcg/kg/min; titrated according to MAP or SVR.
- Can be used alone if CO is satisfactory or in combination with an inotrope (e.g. dobutamine/milrinone) if CO is compromised.
- Risk of arterial conduit vasospasm and a reduction in renal/splanchnic blood flow particularly at higher doses.

Vasopressin
- Endogenous peptide hormone.
- Activity at V1, V2, V3, and oxytocin-type receptors (OTR).

Dose-dependent CVS effects
- Vasoconstriction (V1$_a$) characterizes its clinical effect.
- Relative sparing of pulmonary, coronary, and cerebral circulations.

Splanchnic, skeletal muscle, and cutaneous vessels are particularly affected. Impact on CO is dependent on increases in SVR and reflex changes in HR.

Clinical indications
- Shock (vasodilatory, e.g. vasoplegic syndrome).

Clinical use
- Dosing: 0.01–0.1U/min; commonly 0.04U/min.
- Effects relatively preserved during hypoxia and acidosis.
- Reduces splanchnic blood flow more than noradrenaline and may precipitate myocardial ischaemia at higher doses.
- Often introduced in the context of escalating noradrenaline requirements. Maintains vascular tone when noradrenaline sensitivity is reduced.

Vasodilators

Glyceryl trinitrate
- Vascular smooth muscle relaxation via ↑ cGMP production.

Dose-dependent CVS effects
- Vasodilatation (venous > arterial).
- ↓ preload results in a fall in CO, MVO$_2$, and a modest reduction in MAP. Higher dosing results in a fall in SVR and MAP.

Clinical indications
- Hypertension.
- Acute DHF with pulmonary oedema.
- Myocardial ischaemia.

Clinical use
- Dosing: 1–10mg/hour; titrated upwards according to MAP.
- Although potentially beneficial in the treatment of pulmonary hypertension its use is limited by falls in SVR/MAP.
- Beneficial effects on myocardial ischaemia are primarily due to reductions in MVO$_2$ rather than coronary vasodilatation.
- Tachyphylaxis may occur with prolonged infusion.

Sodium nitroprusside
- Smooth muscle relaxation via release of nitric oxide, increasing cGMP.

Dose-dependent CVS effects
- Vasodilatation (arterial and venous).
- SVR is reduced. CO is maintained or ↑.

Clinical indications
- Hypertension secondary to ↑ SVR.
- Acute DHF.

Clinical use

- Dosing: 0.1–2mcg/kg/min; titrated according to MAP.
- Commonly added to GTN for treatment of resistant hypertension.
- Potential for rebound increases in SVR/MAP on withdrawal.
- Cyanide toxicity is dose and duration dependent and results in tissue hypoxia despite an adequate PaO_2.

Inhaled nitric oxide

- Vascular smooth muscle relaxation via ↑ cGMP.

Dose-dependent effects

- Pulmonary vasodilatation.
- Reduced PVR/RV afterload and improved V/Q matching. Rapidly inactivated by haemoglobin minimizing systemic effects.

Clinical indications

- Pulmonary hypertension and/or RV dysfunction with potential reversibility, e.g. following cardiac transplant, mitral valve surgery.
- ARDS with refractory hypoxaemia.

Clinical use

- Initial dose: 20ppm, with subsequent reduction to achieve minimum effective dose (usually 1–5ppm).
- Titrated according to pulmonary artery pressure measurements.
- Administered via inspiratory limb of a primed ventilator circuit to minimize nitrogen dioxide levels
- Potential for rebound pulmonary hypertension when weaning dose; sildenafil can be used as an adjunct to withdrawal.
- Improvements in PaO_2 in ARDS are not sustained.
- No studies have shown that its use reduces mortality.

Mechanical circulatory support: extracorporeal life support

Mechanical support of the circulation can be lifesaving. Intra-aortic balloon pump (IABP) counterpulsation has long been used as an effective form of circulatory support post cardiotomy; however, it has limitations in advanced circulatory failure. The IABP's main mechanism of action is augmentation of the diastolic myocardial perfusion pressure and reduction in afterload. The improvement in cardiac function often allows weaning of inotropes and the avoidance of harm from their deleterious effects. IABP may be ineffective if cardiac function is profoundly impaired and has the disadvantage that the patient is confined to bed. Short-term ventricular assist devices (VADS) provide full circulatory support which can bridge the patient to either recovery, decision, or transplantation. Where recovery or transplantation is not anticipated in a period of 28 days but is likely to occur, a long-term VAD may be used. Extracorporeal membrane oxygenation (ECMO) may be used for cardiorespiratory support and has a place in the management of both children and adults. The indications, contraindications, and management of these devices are considered in this section.

Intra-aortic balloon pump counterpulsation

IABPs inflate in diastole which augments the diastolic pressure and improves myocardial oxygen supply, deflation on the R wave immediately before systole decreases afterload, and myocardial oxygen demand (Figs 27.1 and 27.2). The improvement in this supply-demand balance improves ischaemic myocardial failure and systemic perfusion.

The commonly used indications for an IABP are:
- Myocardial 'stunning' after cardiac surgery
- Refractory unstable angina awaiting CABG
- Refractory ischaemic ventricular arrhythmias
- The complications of acute MI:
  - Acute severe mitral regurgitation
  - Ventricular septal defect (VSD)
- The unstable primary PCI patient
- Refractory ventricular failure.

Contraindications
- Severe aortic regurgitation
- Severe calcific aorto-iliac disease and/or peripheral vascular disease
- Disease of the descending aorta (aortic coarctation or aneurysm)
- Sheathless insertion in severe obesity.

Potential risks and complications
- Ischaemic limb
- Bleeding from the insertion site
- Aorta perforation or dissection
- Retroperitoneal bleeding
- Patient confined to bed and <45° head up
- Infection risk particularly with femoral cannulation

- Limb ischaemia
- Thrombocytopenia
- Balloon leak
- Compartment syndrome.

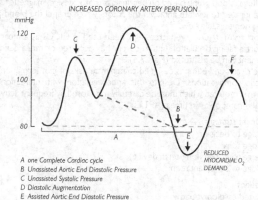

INCREASED CORONARY ARTERY PERFUSION

A one Complete Cardiac cycle
B Unassisted Aortic End Diastolic Pressure
C Unassisted Systolic Pressure
D Diastolic Augmentation
E Assisted Aortic End Diastolic Pressure
F Reduced Systolic Pressure

REDUCED MYOCARDIAL O₂ DEMAND

Figure 27.1 IABP pressure tracing showing diastolic augmentation. Courtesy of MAQUET Cardiac Assist Division.

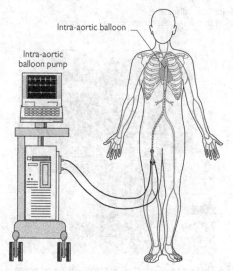

Intra-aortic balloon

Intra-aortic balloon pump

Figure 27.2 Diagram demonstrating an IABP *in situ*. Courtesy of MAQUET Cardiac Assist Division.

Short-term ventricular assist devices

Short-term VADs are used to support a failing circulation for up to 28 days. The commonest device in use currently in the UK is the Levotronix CentriMag® (Fig. 27.3) which is licensed for 28 days. The CentriMag® is a centrifugal blood pump based on bearingless motor design, magnetic forces are generated to levitate and spin the rotors which propel the blood producing non pulsatile flow.

Short-term VADs have increasingly been used in CICUs as a means to support a failing circulation until recovery has occurred or more definitive treatment can be instituted (Fig. 27.4).

The circuit and pump is designed to minimize risks of clot formation and embolic complications. Despite this anticoagulation with unfractionated heparin is required which must be carefully monitored by frequent activated partial thromboplastin times (APTTs).

Treatment strategy
- Bridge to decision
- Bridge to recovery
- Bridge to bridge (long-term device)
- Bridge to transplantation.

Indications
- Dilated cardiomyopathy:
  - Ischaemic
  - Myocarditis
  - Peripartum
- Post cardiotomy
- Congenital heart disease
- Primary graft failure post cardiac transplantation.

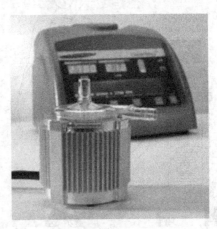

Figure 27.3 The Levitronix CentriMag®. Reprinted with the permission of Thoratec Corporation.

Characteristics of the Levotronix CentriMag®
- Flows up to 9.9L/min
- No seals or bearings, one moving part
- Magnetically levitated impeller
- Licensed for 30 days
- Cost-effective
- Mobility limited.

Different treatment modalities
- Left VAD
- Right VAD
- Bi-VAD
- ECMO.

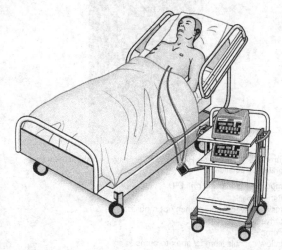

Figure 27.4 A patient with a short-term ventricular assist device. Reprinted with the permission of Thoratec Corporation.

Cannulation options

LVAD
- Inflow cannula:
  - Left atrium (via right upper pulmonary vein)
  - Ventricular apex
- Outflow cannula:
  - Ascending aorta
  - Descending aorta.

RVAD
- Outflow cannula from right atrium
- Inflow cannula to pulmonary artery.

Long-term ventricular assist devices

The main indication for long-term VADs in the UK is bridge to transplantation. Worldwide as the survival on VADs has improved, the use of long-term VADs for destination therapy has ↑.

Indications
- Bridge to transplant
- Bridge to recovery.

Types of long VADS (Fig. 27.5)
- 1st generation: pulsatile displacement pumps
- 2nd generation: continuous flow by rotating impellers
- 3rd generation: centrifugal miniaturized to size of D battery.

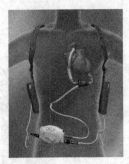

Figure 27.5 The Thoratec HeartMate II®. Reprinted with the permission of Thoratec Corporation.

Components of a long-term LVAD
- Battery pack
- Mains power module when not mobilizing
- Drive line
- Pump
- Inflow cannula from LV apex to pump
- Outflow cannula form pump usually to ascending aorta.

Clinical issues of a long-term LVAD
- Requires functioning RV
- Anticoagulation with warfarin to INR 1.5–2.5
- Battery life 4 hours
- Mobilization possible
- Home discharge is the norm
- Resuscitation:
  • No CPR
  • *Always defibrillate a shockable rhythm*
- Complicates surgical procedure for heart transplantation.

Complications in the early postoperative period in ICU
- Bleeding can be a major problem:
  • The causes are surgical, liver dysfunction, residual anticoagulation, and inflammatory-induced coagulopathy and platelet dysfunction.

- Early intervention to stop haemorrhage is important.
- Surgical reopening is common.
- Anticoagulation should be restarted cautiously once bleeding is controlled.
- Right heart failure:
  - May be due to RV myocardial dysfunction, ventricular interdependence, and ↑ afterload.
  - Excessive blood product administration may elevate the PVR and increase RV overload.
  - RV may be impaired due to underlying aetiology of heart failure.
  - Short-term RVAD hay be required.
  - RV failure may contribute to the 'suck down effect' where the walls of the left ventricle collapse onto the outflow cannula.
- Hypovolaemia may result in poor pump flow due to lack of venous return.
- Respiratory failure.
- Hepto-renal dysfunction.

Long-term complications

The survival at 2 years of patients who were NYHA IIIb or IV and ineligible for transplantation and treated with a continuous flow pump for destination therapy was 58% at 2 years. Complications were common and tended to be infection, bleeding or thromboembolic related.

- Stroke 18%:
  - Ischaemic
  - Haemorrhagic
- Sepsis 36%:
  - Drive line infection
  - Pump and pocket infection
  - Non-LVAD infection
- Pump replacement 9%
- Right heat failure 20%
- Renal and hepatic failure.

ECMO

Extracorporeal life support can be used for cardiorespiratory support (veno-arterial (V-A) ECMO) or respiratory support (veno-venous (V-V) ECMO). In the circuit, generally centrifugal pumps have replaced roller pumps. Compared to CPB, in ECMO a membrane oxygenator designed for long-lasting use is inserted into the circuit. The circuit is simplified to minimize the risk of clotting and inflammatory activation so there is no cardiotomy reservoir.

V-A ECMO

V-A ECMO can be used as 'crash and burn' resuscitative option in patients with acute cardiogenic shock. The technique allows assessment of neurological function and the potential for end-organ recovery prior to embarking on a long-term VAD. It is commonly used in paediatric cardiac surgery for post cardiotomy failure.

- Can be introduced open or percutaneously.
- Femoral arterial cannulation is popular for percutaneous option.

- Venous cannulation is achieved directly from the right atrium or percutaneously via the right internal jugular or femoral veins.

Risks and complications
- Air embolism
- Bleeding
- Thrombotic risk
- Stroke
- Ischaemic limbs
- Haemolysis
- Infection
- Immobility.

V-V ECMO
V-V ECMO is used to allow resting of the lungs in patients with severe respiratory failure. It has been used mainly in neonatal and paediatrics. The duration of support is usually 1–2 weeks.

RDS in the adult population has a mortality in excess of 50%. The CESAR study has demonstrated benefits from specialist ECMO centres in the management of these patients.

Cannulation is by percutaneous cannulation of a major vein (internal jugular and/or femoral) with fluoroscopic (or TOE) guidance. Recent bicaval two-stage cannula (Avalon cannula) can be introduced via the IJV.

The indications and outcomes of ECMO are collected by the ELSO registry. In adults, survival with respiratory V-V ECMO support are better than cardiac V-A ECMO at 55% vs 39% at discharge.

Table 27.1 ECLS Registry report

	Total Patients	Survived ECLS		Survived to DC or Transfer	
Neonatal					
Respiratory	24,770	20,951	85%	18,558	75%
Cardiac	4,375	2,649	61%	1,723	39%
ECPR	694	438	63%	270	39%
Pediatric					
Respiratory	5,009	3,251	65%	2,785	56%
Cardiac	5,423	3,468	64%	2,609	48%
ECPR	1,347	720	53%	539	40%
Adult					
Respiratory	2,620	1,655	63%	1,428	55%
Cardiac	1,680	894	53%	660	39%
ECPR	591	225	38%	173	29%
Total	46,509	34,251	74%	28,745	62%

Data from Extracorporeal Life Support Organization.

Respiratory aetiology of patients treated with ECMO

- Meconium aspiration in neonates
- Viral pneumonitis including influenza and H1N1
- Other pneumonias
- Respiratory distress syndrome
- Trauma including postoperative.

Indications for adult ECMO in the CESAR study

- Age 18–65 years
- Severe respiratory failure but potentially reversible
- Failed conventional management
- Murray score >3.0 or pH< 7.2
- Early referral <7 days with peak inspiratory pressure >30cmH$_2$O and FiO$_2$ >0.8.
- No contraindication to heparin.

Circuit requirements

- Suitable PMP oxygenators include the Maquet Quadrox D® and the Medos Hi-Lite® 7000.
- Centrifugal pump, ideally of modern design such as the Levitronix or Maquet Rotaflow®.
- An ultrasonic flowmeter.
- Monitor pre- and post-membrane pressures.
- Monitor venous drainage (inlet) pressure.
- No venous reservoir.
- No additional connections to reduce risk of air embolism or bleeding.
- High-flow stop-cocks on the drainage and return lines to allow insertion of a bridge.

Targets on V-V ECMO

- Protective lung ventilation:
  - FiO$_2$ 30%, PIP 20–25, PEEP 10–15, rate 10.
- Pressure controlled ventilation or BIPAP.
- Target oxygenation PaO$_2$ 6–8kPa adjusted with ECMO circuit flow.
- PaCO$_2$ 4–6kPa by adjusting sweep gas flow through oxygenator.
- Unfractionated heparin is infused to maintain an ACT at ~180–200 seconds or an APTT ratio of 2–3. These targets depend on the type of ACT machine and local policies.
- Maintain HB at 120–140g/L.

Extracorporeal lung support ECLS

Novalung®

The Novalung® is a new pumpless extracorporeal membrane which efficiently removed CO$_2$ and also improves oxygenation but less efficiently. Indications are ventilator refractory respiratory failure with predominant hypercapnia and respiratory acidosis. There is a developing role in the management of lung transplant graft dysfunction, ARDS, and pneumonias. Generally the left femoral artery and right femoral vein are cannulated percutaneously.

Contraindications
- Heparin allergy or heparin-induced thrombocytopenia
- Cardiogenic shock
- Small femoral artery or occlusive vascular disease.

Technical aspects
- Polymethyl pentene diffusion membrane surface area $1.3m^2$
- Blood flow 0.5–4.5L/min
- Max oxygen flow 15L/min
- 240mL filling volume
- Max. pressure 200mmHg
- Pressure drop at 2.5L/min is 11mmHg
- Maintain MAP at 70–90mmHg as the flow is pressure dependant. Administer noradrenalin if necessary
- Heparin-coated system allows minimal anticoagulation
- Infuse heparin to activated clotting time (ACT) 150–170 or APPT 40–50 seconds
- Check ACT and/or APPT regularly
- Check pulses and clinical perfusion of legs hourly.

Further reading

Peek GJ, Mugford M, Tiruvoipati R, Wilson A, Allen E, Thalanany MM, *et al.* Efficacy and economic assessment of conventional ventilatory support versus extracorporeal membrane oxygenation for severe adult respiratory failure (CESAR): a multicentre randomised controlled trial. *Lancet* 2009;374(9698):1351–63.

Slaughter MS, Rogers JG, Milano CA, Russell SD, Conte JV, Feldman D, *et al.* (2009). Advanced heart failure treated with continuous-flow left ventricular assist device. *NEJM* 2009;361(23):2241–51.

Epicardial pacing

Introduction

Many patients require a short period of pacing after separation from CPB until the normal conduction pathways recover from the rigors of cardioplegia, cooling, and handling of heart. Some patients need it for longer and there may be an eventual need for a permanent pacemaker due to complications of surgery. The majority of patients never require pacing and it is difficult to predict which patients may need pacing. So, most surgeons implant ventricular wires (at least one) in all patients while some do so only when patients required pacing immediately prior to chest closure. Should a patient with a single ventricular wire require pacing a wire is placed under the skin and the pacing circuit completed by attaching the ventricular wire to the negative terminal of the pacing box.

Indications for postoperative pacing:
- Asystole or cardiac standstill
- Complete heart block or type II second-degree heart block
- Bradyarrhythmias (rate control better than with pharmacological intervention)
- Nodal or junctional rhythms
- To restore AV mechanical synchrony
- Sinus arrests
- Prophylaxis against AF
- High-rate burst pacing for control of atrial flutter
- Following heart transplantation.

General principles

When there is endogenous depolarization of the ventricle, this is more mechanically efficient because of the coordinated ventricular contraction. Every effort should be made not to initiate ventricular pacing by first trying atrial pacing. Therefore, atrial wires will be preferable when patients are likely to require pacing, advantages being:

- 25% increase in CO with atrial or AV sequential pacing
- Effect more pronounced in low ejection fraction
- ↑ LV filling in ventricular hypertrophy, ↓ LV compliance—diastolic dysfunction or ischemia.

Informal convention for wires:

- Wires exiting right of sternum—atrial
- Wires exiting left of sternum—ventricular
- Atrial cables—blue tag
- Ventricular cables—white tag

Removal of wires:

- After return of normal coagulation
- Gentle traction and dislodgement by heart contractions
- Excessive resistance—cut close to skin, allowing ends to retract
- Observe patient for few hours—risk of tamponade
- Monitor ECG as risk of arrhythmias.

Consider permanent pacemaker when there is pacemaker dependence after 7 days. Common indications:

- Complete heart block
- Sinus node dysfunction
- Slow ventricular rate with atrial fibrillation
- 2nd-degree Mobitz type II block.

Pacing modes

These are described using the NBG codes, of which only the first three are relevant in temporary epicardial pacing (Table 28.1).

Table 28.1 Pacing modes

I	II	III
Chamber paced	Chamber sensed	Response to sensing
0: none	0: none	0: none
A: atrium	A: atrium	T: triggered
V: ventricle	V: ventricle	I: inhibited
D: dual (A+V)	D: dual (A+V)	D: dual (T+I)

The pacing modes frequently used are as follows.

Single chamber pacing modes

AOO

Atrial asynchronous mode used in stable bradycardia with inappropriate sensing (electrocautery) and intact AV node conduction. Not in atrial tachycardia, flutter, fibrillation or AV nodal block.

VOO

Ventricular asynchronous mode used in bradycardia without reliable AV conduction and when use of electrocautery is causing inappropriate sensing. Also in an emergency as a rapid access function.

AAI

In the atrial demand mode the endogenous atrial depolarization is sensed and an impulse delivered if there is none detected in a cycle determined by the set rate. Used with an endogenous atrial rhythm and intact AV conduction. Not in atrial tachycardia, flutter, fibrillation, or AV nodal block.

VVI

The ventricular demand mode is similar to AAI, but the chamber involved is the ventricle. This is used when there is bradycardia with AV block, atrial flutter, AF, or sick sinus syndrome. Also, when atrial wires are avoided to decrease possible complications when need for pacing is predicted to be of short duration or to suppress ectopic beats with overdrive pacing. Downside is the loss of atrial contribution to ventricular filling.

DDD

This is the commonest and most useful mode when both atrial and ventricular wires are in place. The other dual chamber pacing modes are DOO, DVI, and DDI and will not be discussed in this section.

In DDD mode both chambers are sensed and paced in sequence. Firstly, as in AAI, if no endogenous atrial depolarization is detected in a predetermined rate-dependent cycle an impulse is delivered to the atrium. The pacemaker then waits for a ventricular impulse in response to atrial pacing or an endogenous atrial depolarization and delivers an impulse if none is detected within the cycle. This mode is used in all indications for pacing. There is a risk of ventricular tracking of atrial tachyarrhythmias which is off-set by setting a 'maximum tracking rate'.

Antitachycardia modes

Many of the commonly occurring postsurgical tachyarrhythmias can be treated by overdrive pacing. VF or VT may occur during the process and so needs adequate preparation:

AV junctional tachycardia

This is treated by using overdrive pacing of either atria (AAI or AOO) or sequential AV pacing (DDD or DOO). The cardiac rate is captured by pacing at 120% of the intrinsic rate and then gradually reduced, establishing stable sinus rhythm.

Paroxysmal re-entrant supraventricular tachycardia

Can be treated as described earlier or by using 'under-drive' pacing (at less than the supraventricular tachycardia (SVT) rate) if the pacing spike induces a refractory period in the re-entrant loop and abolishes it.

Atrial flutter

Over-drive pacing as previously described is effective in type I flutter with rates <320–340 but not in type II with higher rates.

Failed SVT reversion with rapid ventricular response

In this situation rapid atrial pacing at rates up to 800 beats/min may induce AF and may be preferable if the AV block is high enough to have a slower ventricular response. Sometimes this manoeuvre may induce reversion to sinus rhythm.

Ventricular tachycardia

Overdrive or underdrive pacing may terminate VT but remains a risky manoeuvre as it can precipitate VF.

Troubleshooting

Failure to pace

This is differentiated from failure to capture by absence of pacing spikes (no electricity at wire tips) on ECG, a slower than set heart rate, and can be due to:
- Lead disconnection
- Lead malfunction (fractured wire)
- Battery depletion
- Over-sensing
- Cross-talk.

Failure to capture

There is presence of pacing spikes on ECG but is not followed by QRS complex or waveform on arterial pressure and pulse oximeter and can be due to:
- A low pacemaker output (mA)
- A high stimulation threshold
- Pacing wire displacement from myocardium
- ↑ resistance due to fibrosis
- Myocardial ischemia
- Electrolyte imbalance
- Medications like β-blockers, verapamil, lidocaine, sotalol, flecainide, or propafenone.

Manoeuvres which may be helpful:
- Increasing pacemaker output
- Correction of exacerbating factors listed earlier
- Reversing polarity of bipolar pacing wires
- Changing to unipolar pacing with subcutaneous return pacing wire
- Temporary transvenous or oesophageal pacing if threshold progressively increasing
- Transcutaneous pacing in an emergency.

Failure to sense

This must be distinguished from normal pacemaker function with inappropriate settings. Check sensing threshold (see 🕮 Mandatory checks, p. 310).

Cross-talk

This occurs in dual-chamber pacing modes when the atrial pacing spike is sensed by the ventricular wire and inhibits ventricular output.
  Manoeuvres which may be helpful:
- Reduce sensitivity (mV)
- Reduce pacing output (mA)

Mandatory checks

The stimulation and sensing thresholds should be checked at the earliest opportune moment and then daily in addition to a battery check. Stimulation threshold checked in all patients and sensing threshold once an intrinsic rhythm has been established. The underlying rhythm should be checked regularly by turning down the pacing rate and letting the endogenous rhythm to emerge, thereby assessing ongoing need for pacing.

Stimulation threshold

This is the minimum output (mA) needed to consistently capture the heart.

Method of assessing

- Set rate at 10 above patient's intrinsic rate (if established)
- Decrease pacemaker output slowly until loss of capture
- Increase output until there is steady capture
- This is stimulation threshold
- Set output twice stimulation threshold.

Sensing threshold

This is the least sensitive setting (biggest mV value) at which the pacemaker can detect a heartbeat.

Method of assessing

- Set rate to 10 below patient's intrinsic rate.
- Set ventricular output to 0.1mA (this prevents an inadvertent 'R-on-T'-induced ventricular tachyarrhythmia).
- Press menu key until the menu is displayed (see Fig. 28.1 for a Medtronic pacemaker box menu).
- Highlight V sensitivity.
- Decrease sensitivity (increase mV value) until sense indicator stops flashing.
- Increase until it starts flashing again—sensing threshold.
- Set sensitivity dial to one half the mV value.

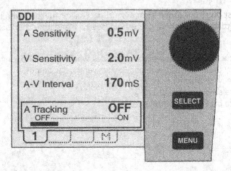

Figure 28.1 Pacemaker box menu. With kind permission from Medtronic.

Complications of pacing wires

- Bleeding and haematoma
- Tamponade
- Myocardial damage
- Perforation
- Infection
- Disruption of coronary anastomosis
- Inadvertent disconnection of the lead system
- Asystole following abrupt cessation of pacing
- Ventricular tachyarrhythmias due to inappropriate pacing
- Muscle and nerve stimulation.

Further reading

Reade MC. Temporary epicardial pacing after cardiac surgery: a practical review: Part 1: General considerations in the management of epicardial pacing. *Anaesthesia* 2007;62:264–71.

Reade MC. Temporary epicardial pacing after cardiac surgery: a practical review: Part 2: Selection of epicardial pacing modes and troubleshooting. *Anaesthesia* 2007;62:364–73.

Sedation and pain relief

Introduction

After cardiac surgery, patients require a short period of sedation or symptom control to minimize oxygen consumption while they re-establish their normal physiology. This return of patient homeostasis includes re-establishing normothermia, normal coagulation, fluid balance, and vasomotor control.

Patients after minimally invasive and off-pump procedures can be considered for early extubation but still have to be supported with a satisfactory analgesic protocol.

The environment in ICU is associated with many factors that can affect patient comfort, safety, and overall experience. Pain, anxiety, and sleep disruption may disrupt neurocognitive function and are contributing factors for the development of delirium and post-traumatic stress disorder (PTSD).

This chapter describes the pharmacology of sedative and analgesic drugs, modern concepts and pathways, and patient assessment.

Principles of sedation

We must differentiate short-term sedation in the uncomplicated patient from long-term sedation in unstable patients who develop critical illness. The following aspects should be considered:

- Short-term sedation is mainly protocol driven and aims at timely extubation using short-acting agents.
- There has been a shift from hypnosis-driven sedation to a more opioid-based technique.
- Good sedation allows symptom control and achieves a calm and approachable patient.
- Sedation in unstable and critically ill patients needs to be adapted with regard to its impact on haemodynamics and organ dysfunction.
- Longer exposure to sedation often leads to adaption processes such as tolerance to opioids or tachyphylaxis to benzodiazepines.
- Sedation protocols should have targets and allow for sedation breaks.

Principles of pain relief

Experience of postoperative pain is often complex and multifactorial. It depends not only on somatic but also on emotional stress. Modern concepts of postoperative analgesia are based on

- Multimodal approaches including local anaesthetics
- Favourable pharmacokinetics and pharmacodynamics
- Good ability to titrate to patient's requirements
- No or minimal adjustments in patients with organ dysfunction
- Pharmaco-economics.

Further reading

Schweikert WD, Kress JP. Strategies to optimise analgesia and sedation. *Crit Care* 2008;12(Supp. 3):S6.
Sessler CN, Varney K. Patient-focused sedation and analgesia in the ICU. *Chest* 2008;133:552–65.
Tonner PH, Weiler N, Paris A, Scholz J. Sedation and analgesia in the intensive care unit. *Curr Opin Anaesthesiol* 2003;16:113–21.

Patient assessment

Although it appears obvious to identify patients who are comfortable and differentiate them from those who are not, it can be difficult to quantify and scale these conditions and make these measurements the basis of decision-making and intervention.

Assessment tools

The Richmond Agitation-Sedation Scale (RASS)

This is a useful and validated 10-point scoring scale developed in a collaborative way by critical care doctors, nurses, pharmacists, and physiotherapists. Now widely used clinically and for research (see Table 15.3).

Confusion Assessment Method for ICU (CAM-ICU)

This scoring is designed to explore delirious patients. It is based on a combined assessment of the mental status beyond the influence of pharmacological sedation. CAM-ICU includes:
- Level of inattention
- Altered level of consciousness
- Degree of disorganized thinking.

Electroencephalogram

Although processed EEG parameters, like BIS or entropy as well as evoked potentials, have been successfully used to titrate general anaesthetics, they have proven less useful in distinguishing and reflecting the more subtle changes of ICU sedation. The use of EEG is still recommended to identify:
- Seizures and focal epilepsy
- Burst suppression pattern during hypothermia
- Adequate level of hypnosis in the paralysed patient.

Visual Analogue Scale (VAS)

Traditional instrument to quantify the level of pain and discomfort. Normally used as an 11-point scale with 0=no pain and 10 (100) representing the worst imaginable pain. Although the VAS is still widely used, there are a lot of shortcomings that limit its usefulness. The VAS:
- Is operator biased
- Has huge situational variability
- Poor agreement between patients
- Traditionally widely used in studies
- Helpful to follow-up individuals

Functional capacity

A more meaningful description of the effectiveness of analgesia is the extent of functional recovery that a patient is able to achieve at any given stage. Examples of functional capacity after cardiac surgery are:
- Productive chest clearance
- Mobilization
- Walking distance
- Walking on stairs.

Aims and strategies

Providing patient comfort and safety

This should include minimizing pain and facilitating tube tolerance, minimizing anxiety, and avoiding adverse effects.

Optimizing patient recovery

This includes faster achievement of recovery goals such as extubation and mobilization, but also allows more effective physiological and functional recovery, e.g. intensive chest physiotherapy.

Further reading

Haenggi M, Ypparila-Wolters H, Hauser K, Caviezel C, Takala J, Korhonen I, et al. Intra- and inter-individual variation of BIS-index and Entropy during controlled sedation with midazolam/remifentanil and dexmedetomidine/remifentanil in healthy volunteers: an interventional study. *Crit Care* 2009;13:R20.

Sessler CN, Gosnell MS, Grap MJ, Brophy GM, O'Neal PV, Keane KA, et al. The Richmond Agitation-Sedation Scale. *Am J Respir Crit Care Med* 2002;166:1338–44.

Vanderbilt University Medical Center. Delirium resources. Available at: 𝒥ⓑ <http://www.mc.vanderbilt.edu/icudelirium/assessment.html>

Pharmacology

There are only a limited number of drugs that qualify as candidates for sedation and analgesia for the cardiac patient. Most drugs work synergistically when used together, so lower doses/concentrations of each component is advisable.

Opioids

Morphine

Popular and effective opioid that also has sedative characteristics. Mainly used intravenously by nurse-controlled boluses or patient-controlled analgesia. Unsuitable for long-term exposure due to high variability in pharmacodynamics and metabolism. Its active metabolite is morphine-6-glucuronate. Absorption of subcutaneous morphine can be difficult to predict in poorly perfused patients. Morphine is emetogenic and impairs gut motility.

Alfentanil

Short-acting opioid that is given by IV infusion. Shallow dose–response curve allows it to be used in spontaneously breathing patients. Usually rapid recovery when infusion is weaned. However, recovery can be affected in genetically determined slow metabolizers across the cytochrome P450 pathway (about 25% of Caucasian patients).

Remifentanil

Ultra-short-acting fentanyl congener with context-sensitive half-time of only 3–4 minutes. Elimination independent of organ dysfunction. Increasingly used for short-term postoperative sedation until and after extubation. Easy to titrate. This can be further improved by using remifentanil as target-controlled infusion (TCI) for which it is licensed.

Pethidine (meperidine)

A relatively old phenylpiperidine with characteristics similar to morphine. Today mainly used to control postoperative shivering against which it is highly effective.

Sedatives/hypnotics

Propofol

Popular hypnotic that is easy to titrate and rapid to recover from. Can be administered as TCI. When used for long-term sedation, triglyceride levels should be checked regularly. Reports of severe lactic acidosis and hyper-metabolism in critically ill children and adults (propofol infusion syndrome (PIS)). However, PIS seems to be rare in daily practice and associated with exposure to unreasonably high doses.

Midazolam

Widely used short-acting benzodiazepine that acts as sedative, anxiolytic, amnesic, and anticonvulsant. Sedative and respiratory depressant characteristics are potentiated with concomitant use of opioids. Elderly patients are often highly sensitive to midazolam and recover very slowly. Drug may accumulate after long exposure and in patients with organ dysfunction.

Clonidine

α-2 adrenoceptor agonist that is highly effective for symptom control in agitated patients and for alcohol withdrawal. Increasingly used for long-term ICU patients to wean off the ventilator. Bradycardia and hypotension can occur if drug is loaded too quickly. Should not be used in patients on high doses of inotropes.

Dexmedetomidine

Highly selective α-2 adrenoceptor agonist. Recent studies have shown non-inferiority compared to propofol and midazolam. Experience in cardiac ICU is still limited. Licensed in the UK since 2011 for sedation of adult ICU patients requiring sedation level no deeper than arousal in response to verbal stimulation (corresponding to RASS score 0 to −3).

Antipsychotics/NMDA-antagonists

Haloperidol

Neuroleptic agent that is now considered as first choice for treatment of delirium. Given in increasing increments to control symptoms. Similar to droperidol, it can alter the QT interval and trigger torsade de pointes arrhythmia in vulnerable patients.

Ketamine

NMDA-receptor antagonist that modulates short- and long-term pain. Reduces development of hyperalgesia after opioid exposure. Current evidence suggests ultra-low doses of around 0.05mg/kg/hour. Extrapyramidal side effects when used in higher doses. Available as isomeric S-(+)-ketamine in some countries.

Further reading

Baltali S, Turkoz A, Bozdogan N, Demirturk OS, Baltali M, Turkoz R, et al. The efficacy of intravenous patient-controlled remifentanil versus morphine anesthesia after coronary artery surgery. *J Cradiothorac Vasc Anesth* 2009;23:170–4.

Riker RR, Shehabi Y, Bokesch PM, Ceraso D, Wisemandle W, Koura F, *et al*. Dexmedetomidine vs midazolam for sedation of critically ill patients. *JAMA* 2009;301:489–99.

Clinical protocols

Most institutions have developed standards, protocols, and care bundles with regard to the practical aspects of sedation and analgesia. In many cardiac critical care units the default strategy is executed and managed by nurses and nurse practitioners.

Although there is no clear evidence which sedative drugs or drug combinations are superior over others, modern practice is mainly influenced by the aim of reduced length of stay in ICU and avoiding unnecessary long ventilation times. The choice of drugs will then inevitably be influenced by the best available to achieve these goals.

To allow a predictable and patient-focused pain management, a single analgesic pathway should be favoured that can be modified in specific patients that need additional attention. The availability of an Acute Pain Service is helpful in managing patients with complex pain issues or even pre-existing algesic syndromes.

Any technique or pathway for both sedation and analgesia should be designed to:
• Be simple and predictable to administer
• Be safe across a variety of patient groups
• Have little or no interaction with concurrent treatment.

An example protocol

Routine cardiac postoperative patient after surgery with CPB:
• On propofol and remifentanil (preferably TCI) on arrival in ICU.
• Stop propofol when warm, haemodynamically stable, and no major blood loss.
• Reduce remifentanil to allow spontaneous ventilation but still provide tolerance of ETT.
• Extubate patient when awake and cooperative.

Pain management

There are two major stages that characterize the analgesic requirements of a postoperative cardiac patient. These can be described as the early postoperative phase and the later step-down analgesia phase.

Although it is generally desirable to convert the patient to oral analgesia as soon as possible, this can be confounded by delayed GI adsorption and motility or by issues around nausea.

Early postoperative phase
• Manage with IV morphine or continue remifentanil infusion (see example protocol). Allow regular IV paracetamol supplements.
• Convert to potent oral opioid analgesics like oxycodone (combined fast- and slow-release formulations) and oral paracetamol when GI adsorption is deemed satisfactory.
• NSAIDs only in suitable patients. These drugs can interfere with coagulation, renal function, and gastric mucosal integrity. Contraindicated in patients with endocoronary stents.

Step-down analgesia
- Switch to composite balanced analgesic drugs, like co-codamol.
- Allow lower potency opioids, like tramadol for rescue PRN.
- NSAIDs in suitable patients.

Wound management

Sternal wounds

Management of the uncomplicated sternal wound

- Minimize hypothermia, pain, hypovolaemia, and vasoconstriction.
- Optimize haemodynamics.
- Leave the original dressing undisturbed for first 24 hours to allow adequate time for skin edges to seal. Expose non-draining incisions after 24–48 hours to promote wound healing.
- Practice meticulous hand washing and aseptic wound.
- Splint the entire rib cage while suctioning or coughing to minimize wound stress.

Sternal wound complications

- *Mediastinal dehiscence*: median sternotomy wound breakdown in the absence of clinical or microbiological evidence of infection.
- *Mediastinal wound infection*: clinical or microbiological evidence of infected presternal tissue and sternal osteomyelitis, with or without mediastinal sepsis and with or without unstable sternum. Subtypes include:
  - *Superficial wound infection*: wound infection confined to the subcutaneous tissue.
  - *Deep wound infection or mediastinitis*: wound infection associated with sternal osteomyelitis with or without infected retrosternal space.

Deep sternal wound infections or mediastinitis can be further subclassified depending on the presence of risk factors, latency of presentation, and response to treatment.

Presentation and diagnosis

Infection may present within 4–5 days of surgery but more commonly patients are readmitted from home or from ward to critical care with discharging sternotomy wound. They may be systemically unwell with signs of sepsis:

- Wound erythema, induration, and warmth
- Excessive pain and tenderness
- Discharge: from sterile colourless fluid to frank, culture positive pus
- Sternal instability in addition to previous points may indicate deep infection
- Tachycardia, fever, shivering, lethargy.

Sternal wound infection may start as a localized area of sternal osteomyelitis, with minimal visible signs followed by sternal separation.

Practice point

Check for sternal instability by gentle bi-manual palpation. Warn the patient that this may be painful.

Investigations
- *Wound swabs or pus*: microscopy, culture, and sensitivity.
- *White cell count, C-reactive protein* (neutrophilia).
- *CXR*:
  - Widened mediastinum or enlarged cardiac silhouette
  - Uni- or bilateral pleural effusion
  - Pulmonary infiltrates.
- *CT scan*: best available non-invasive evaluation. May show cut-through wires, separated sternal halves, substernal or retro cardiac collection, or in late cases mediastinal collection with air fluid levels.

Common pathogens
- *Staphylococcus aureus*: most common
- Coagulase-negative *Staphylococcus*: increasing
- Mixed infections
- Gram-negative pathogens
- Fungi.

Mediastinitis can be diagnosed if at least one of the following is present:
- An organism isolated from culture of mediastinal tissue or fluid.
- Evidence of mediastinitis seen during operation.
- One of the following conditions: chest pain, sternal instability, or fever (>38.8°C), in combination with either purulent discharge from the mediastinum or an organism isolated from blood culture or culture of mediastinal drainage.

Prevention
- Perioperative mupirocin ointment in patients with nasal colonization of *Staphylococcus aureus*.
- Optimum timing of prophylactic antibiotics.
- Meticulous attention to skin preparation and operative technique. Short cardiopulmonary bypass and operation time.
- Control of plasma glucose (4–10mmol/L).

Management

Superficial wound infection
- Incision and effective drainage if there is localization and 'pointing'.
- Thorough inspection and debridement of involved soft tissue. Remove exposed sternal wires if possible (may be necessary to leave *in situ* until sternal integrity is re-established).
- Culture-directed antimicrobial therapy.
- Appropriate dressings (local protocols).
- Vacuum-assisted closure (VAC) device may be useful in more extensive forms of superficial wound infection.

Deep wound infection
- Establish and treat the causative pathogens.
- Mainstay of treatment is surgical revision, including thorough debridement and preparation of the wound for reconstruction. Options include:
  - In the absence of gross infection, primary closure after thorough debridement and sternal fixation (may involve simple plastic surgical techniques such as pectoral advancement flaps).
  - In the presence of gross infection, secondary closure after a period of conventional wound drainage.
  - Treatment with vacuum (VAC) dressing system (both for clean or infected wounds). VAC therapy can be used as a definitive treatment allowing the wound to granulate and heal, or as a prelude to secondary closure.
  - Secondary closure may require plastic surgical techniques.
- General measures:
  - Cover open sternal wounds with sterile dressing to protect from respiratory secretions and drainage contamination. Elevate the head of the bed and cover the chest with waterproof drape when suctioning.
  - Monitor wounds on regular basis. Clear documentation is important: description of wound edges, slough, granulation tissue, and discharge.
  - Monitor closely for cardiovascular and respiratory complications. Sternal instability and pain can reduce respiratory volumes by 50%.
  - Maintain airway clearance (coughing and deep breathing, incentive spirometry, ambulation, repositioning, and postural drainage).
  - Multidisciplinary approach: dieticians, pharmacist, and physiotherapist. Monitor weight, intake of calories, and essential nutrients.
  - Person-centred care (may be a long haul): reassuring manner, eye contact, touch and reality orientation, involvement of family and significant others, adequate sleep, distraction, and relaxation (TV, music).
  - Control of plasma glucose (4–10mmol/L).

VAC dressing
- Open drainage with continuous removal of exudate with simultaneous stabilization of the chest and isolation of the wound.
- Maintains a moist environment and stimulates granulation-tissue formation in combination with an ↑ blood flow in the adjacent tissue.
- Approximates the wound edges and provides a mass filling effect with a low degree of surgical trauma, without establishing a new wound (e.g. abdominal wound in omental flaps).
- Due to sternal stabilization and wound isolation, patients can be mobilized and receive physiotherapy early.

Further reading

Francel TJ. A rational approach to sternal wound complications. *Semin Thorac Cardiovasc Surg* 2004;16(1):81–91.

National Institute for Health and Clinical Excellence. *Surgical Site Infection*. Clinical guideline 74. London: NICE; 2008. Available at: ℞ <http://www.nice.org.uk/CG74>.

Reida M, Oakley EL, Wright JE. Postoperative mediastinitis: classification and management. *Ann Thorac Surg* 1996;61:1030–6.

Saphenous vein site

Management of uncomplicated leg wounds

- After skin closure, dress wound and firmly apply crepe bandage.
- Apply compression stockings for DVT prophylaxis.
- Leave wound intact for first 48 hours unless there is excessive soakage. Redress using sterile dressing till 5th postoperative day after which leave open.
- Early ambulation and physiotherapy.
- Caution in patients with peripheral vascular disease in the application of tight bandages. A regular check of the peripheral pulses must be incorporated into routine postoperative observations.
- NICE guidelines (2007) report a significantly lower rate of wound infection following endoscopic vs open vein harvest.

Leg wound complications

Minor
- Erythema, induration, and cellulitis
- Dermatitis
- Greater saphenous nerve paraesthesia
- Persistent leg swelling
- Seroma and lymphocoele.

Major (requiring surgical intervention)
- Infection
- Non-healing wound
- Wound necrosis
- Limb ischaemia.

Leg wound infections are usually seen after 3–4 days postoperatively and thus may not be seen commonly in intensive care. Many patients are re-admitted after their primary discharge from hospital and the majority can be managed on ward basis with regular debridement and dressing.

Occasionally patients may present to intensive care after surgical intervention for severe, deep rooted, neglected, or aggressive infections, ± vascular procedures directed at underlying peripheral vascular disease. These patients are likely to be in catabolic status due to prolonged effects of infection, possibly with superadded acute sepsis.

Radial artery harvest site

Radial artery wound complications
- Limb ischaemia
- Compartment syndrome
- Infection
- Dysaesthesia.

Ischaemia

With attention to preoperative selection and operative technique, hand ischaemia is a very rare complication of radial artery harvest. Recently, some reports have suggested presence of 'mild hand ischaemia' in around 10% patients which is manifested by exercise intolerance and is thought to arise due to poor ulnar artery flow reserve.

At transfer of patient from theatre, presence of radial artery wound should be noted and capillary refill in fingers should be checked and documented.

In ICU distal ulnar pulse, skin colour, and capillary refill should be checked at regular intervals. If there is any doubt bandaging should be loosened and close observation continued.

Early vascular intervention is paramount if limb salvage is to be successful in true limb ischaemia.

Acute compartment syndrome

This is rare as muscle fascia is usually deliberately left unclosed after radial artery harvest. It is important not to miss the diagnosis as early treatment is paramount. Treatment is by opening the wound and fasciotomy.

Diagnosis of compartment syndrome after radial artery harvest
- High index of suspicion.
- Key early sign is disproportionate pain, especially on movement or stretching.
- Classical signs of pallor, pulselessness, and paralysis are late manifestations.
- In the early phase pulse may be palpable because the systolic pressure is >30mmHg intracompartmental pressure typically associated with the syndrome
- Measurement of the intracompartment pressure especially in patients who are ventilated or obtunded.

Dysaesthesia

Incidence of neurological complications following radial artery harvest has usually been reported to be 5–10% and consists of ↓ thumb strength and dorsal or palmer sensation abnormalities. Most symptoms resolve in the first year after the surgery.

Thoracotomy wounds

- Haematoma and bleeding
- Disruption
- Infection
- Pain (see 📖 Sedation and pain relief, p. 313).

Haematoma and bleeding

Most haematomas are self-limiting and can be managed conservatively. Occasionally, they may be associated with bleeding from wound margins which may not stop despite compression. This may need an additional suture or two, or, in extreme cases, the wound may need to be locally explored to evacuate the haematoma.

Disruption

This varies from a localized area of wound opening to extensive wound disruption involving all the layers of wound. Disruption may or may not be associated with infection.

- Superficial localized area of wound disruption. Swab to rule out infection and leave open to granulate. A clean, non-contaminated, immediately postoperative wound can be closed, but monitor for later development of infection.
- More complete disruptions will require more formal surgical revision. Very rarely, complete disruption of deeper layers of wounds with intact superficial layers can present with surgical emphysema and palpable bulge on coughing.

Infection

Thoracotomy wounds are significantly more painful compared with median sternotomy wounds but infection is less common.

Infection can enter from external sources or from infected pleural space. Usually associated with partial or complete wound disruption. Beware development of 'pus pockets' connected to the main wound by narrow channels. Management follows general principles of debridement followed by granulation or secondary closure, possibly over a drain. For wound infection associated with empyema, 'open tube thoracotomy' can be employed through a separate chest drain to drain the pleural collection. The tube is gradually withdrawn as the empyema pocket shrinks. Development of bronchopleural fistula is a serious complication.

Infection control and prevention

Infection control

Hospital-acquired infections (HAIs) remain a significant cause of morbidity and mortality in the UK. A 1-day prevalence study of European ICUs found that 21% of patients had an ICU-acquired infection. Patients in an ICU setting are more susceptible to HAIs due to underlying illness severity, presence of prosthetic material, e.g. central lines, urinary catheters, and exposure to broad-spectrum antibiotics. The risk of HAIs in ICU patients can be reduced by adherence to basic infection control precautions, prudent antimicrobial prescribing, and care of invasive devices.

Infection control precautions

Infection control precautions can be divided into two main categories:

Standard infection control precautions (SICPs)

SICPs are necessary to reduce the risk of transmission of micro-organisms and should be carried out as a minimum for all patients. They include:

- Hand hygiene
- Use of personal protective equipment (PPE), e.g. gloves, aprons
- Control of the environment
- Management of equipment
- Occupational exposure management
- Management of blood and body fluid spillages
- Appropriate patient placement
- Safe disposal of waste and linen.

Transmission-based precautions (TBPs)

TBPs should be used in addition to standard precautions when a patient is known or suspected to have a specific infection. TBPs will be based on the mode of transmission of the particular agent and can be divided into three main categories:

- Droplet, e.g. influenza, meningococcal disease
- Contact, e.g. *Clostridium difficile*, meticillin-resistant *Staphylococcus aureus* (MRSA)
- Airborne, e.g. *Mycobacterium tuberculosis*, chickenpox.

Not all three categories will necessarily be essential for each particular infectious agent and advice should therefore be sought from local infection control teams.

Hand hygiene

Scrupulous hand hygiene is considered the single most effective measure for the prevention of healthcare-associated infection. Audits of hand hygiene opportunities, however, often reveal poor compliance amongst healthcare workers.

Skin flora can be divided into two types:

- *Transient organisms*—these are picked up from the patient or environment and are not usually part of the normal flora, e.g. MRSA, *Pseudomonas* spp.
- *Resident organisms*—these are organisms such as coagulase-negative staphylococci and *Corynebacterium* spp., i.e. skin flora which are found deep in the dermis and don't tend to cause infection unless introduced during an invasive procedure, e.g. central line insertion.

When to wash?

- Before patient contact
- Before aseptic task
- After body fluid exposure risk
- After patient contact
- After contact with patient surroundings.

In addition to the five key moments in Box 31.1, hand washing should take place after handling food, using the toilet, and when visibly contaminated.

Alcohol hand gel

Alcohol hand gel can be used between episodes of *single* patient care (hygienic hand disinfection). When hands are visibly contaminated soap and water should be used (hygienic hand wash). Alcohol gel is not sufficient for hand hygiene in patients with *Clostridium difficile* as it has no activity against spores.

Surgical hand disinfection

Surgical hand disinfection needs to take place prior to performing surgical or invasive procedures. The hands and forearms must be washed for a minimum of 2 minutes with an antiseptic detergent, e.g. povidone-iodine or chlorhexidine.

Prudent antimicrobial prescribing

All trusts will have antimicrobial management teams who are responsible for the development, implementation, and audit of antibiotic policies. Policies will generally be available for empirical prescribing, surgical prophylaxis, and for organism-specific conditions. Other methods employed to control antibiotic prescribing include:
- Alert antibiotic policies, i.e. antibiotics that can only be prescribed after discussions with a microbiologist or infectious diseases physician.
- IV to oral switch policies.
- Electronic prescribing.
- Automatic stop orders.
- Antibiotic cycling or rotation.

The aim of such interventions is the reduction of antibiotic resistance and the reduction of infections due to resistant organisms such as *Clostridium difficile* and MRSA amongst others.

Clostridium difficile infection (CDI)

Clostridium difficile is an anaerobic Gram-positive rod which was first linked to pseudomembranous colitis in 1978. It is now the most common cause of hospital-acquired diarrhoea and is associated with ↑ morbidity and mortality. In 2008, a new ribotype was recognized following an outbreak in Quebec, Canada. This 027 strain now present in the UK is associated with more severe disease, disease refractory to treatment, and mortality, effects which are due to hyper-production of toxin. Risk factors for CDI in the ICU patient include the use of broad-spectrum antibiotics, proton pump inhibitors (PPIs), prolonged duration of stay, and serious underlying illness.

Reducing the risk of CDI

- Hand hygiene—hands must be washed with soap and water according to the five moments listed in Box 31.1.
- Isolation—patients should be nursed in a single room.
- Use of PPE, e.g. gloves, aprons.
- Enhanced cleaning—the environment should be cleaned twice daily with a chlorine-based detergent.
- Prudent prescribing—prescribe as per local policy. Review need for antibiotics daily. Restrict use of high-risk antibiotics—the 4Cs— Clindamycin, Co-amoxiclav, Cephalosporins, Ciprofloxacin.
- Review need for PPI.

Management of CDI

- Consider stopping antibiotics, PPIs, antimotility agents.
- Implement stool chart—monitor frequency daily.
- Review fluid and electrolytes daily.
- Assess severity of disease. Severity criteria include: colonic dilatation >6cm, creatinine >1.5× baseline, temperature >38.5°C, white cell count >15×10^9 cells/L, immunosuppression:
  - Patients with 0–1 severity markers and non-severe disease should be treated first line with metronidazole 400mg three times a day for 10–14 days.
  - Patients with >2 severity markers should be commenced on oral vancomycin 125mg four times a day for 10–14 days. If ileus is present IV metronidazole should be added.
  - If abdomen is distended or painful a radiological assessment should be undertaken and a surgical review requested.

MRSA

MRSA remains an important nosocomial pathogen and a cause of significant morbidity and mortality in an ICU setting. Cardiothoracic patients will normally undergo preoperative MRSA screening of two or more body sites. Ideally those who test positive should undergo decolonization and have two negative MRSA screens prior to surgery.

Decolonization therapy consists of:

- Nasal application of 2% mupirocin ointment three times daily for 5 days.
- Body washes with agents such as HiBiSCRUB® or Clinisan Advance™.

In an emergency situation where there is no time for eradication, a decolonization regimen should be commenced as soon as possible and surgical antibiotic prophylaxis should consist of antibiotics with activity against MRSA, e.g. glycopeptide ± gentamicin.

Influenza

Influenza is one of the commonest causes of upper respiratory tract infection. Respiratory complications such as viral and bacterial pneumonias are more common in patients with pre-existing heart and lung disease.

In the critical care setting infection control precautions (ICPs) for patients during an influenza pandemic should be implemented on admission and continued for the duration of the illness. These ICPs and other containment measures include:

- Adherence to SICPs and droplet precautions.
- Isolation or cohorting of affected patients.
- Hand hygiene.
- PPE—in addition to gloves and aprons, surgical masks are recommended for close contact (<1m) with a patient. An FFP3 respirator and eye protection are recommended in patients undergoing aerosol generating procedures.
- Exclusion of symptomatic staff and visitors.
- Environmental cleaning.
- Vaccination of patients and staff.

In addition, there are specific precautions which should be taken in relation to respiratory equipment. These include:

- The use of disposable equipment where possible.
- Closed ventilation systems where possible.
- The ventilatory circuit should not be broken unless essential—if a break occurs appropriate PPE for aerosol-generating procedures should be worn.
- All respiratory equipment should have a high efficiency bacterial/viral filter which should be changed in line with manufacturers' recommendations.

Care of devices

Devices such as urinary catheters and peripheral and central venous catheters are associated with an ↑ risk of HAI. In intensive care settings care bundles have been implemented to reduce the number of device-associated HAIs. These bundles are comprised of basic evidence-based procedures grouped together in a single protocol with the aim being to improve patient outcomes. Bundles can be performed during insertion and maintenance of the device. An example of a peripheral venous catheter bundle is as follows;

- Check the PVCs *in situ* are still required.
- Remove PVCs where there is extravasation or inflammation.
- Check PVC dressings are intact.
- Consider removal of PVCs *in situ* >72 hours.
- Perform hand hygiene before and after all PVC procedures.

Further reading

Coia JE, Duckworth GJ, Edwards DI, Farrington M, Fry C, Humphreys H, *et al*. Guidelines for the control and prevention of MRSA in healthcare facilities. *J Hosp Infect*. 2006;63:S1–S44

Department of Health. *Pandemic Influenza. Guidance for Infection Control in Clinical Care*. London: Department of health; 2008. Available at: ✍<http://www.dhsspsni.gov.uk/guidance_for_infection_control_in_critical_care__420kb_.pdf>.

Health Protection Scotland. *PVC Care Bundle*. Available at: ✍ <http://www.hps.scot.nhs.uk/haiic/ic/PVCCareBundle.aspx>.

Vincent JL, Bihari DJ, Suter PM, Bruining HA, White J, Nicolas-Chanoin MH, *et al*. The prevalence of nosocomial infection in intensive care units in Europe. Results of the European Prevalence of Infection in Intensive Care (EPIC) study. *JAMA* 1995;274:639–44.

World Health Organization. *WHO Guidelines on Hand Hygiene in Healthcare*. 2009. Available at: ✍ <http://www.who.int/rpc/guidelines/9789241597906/en/>.

Antimicrobial therapy

Empiric broad-spectrum antimicrobial therapy is started when there is a strong clinical suspicion of infection. This should be de-escalated to narrow-spectrum antimicrobial therapy if culture results permit to reduce the risk of resistant organisms and opportunistic infections, e.g. *Clostridium difficile*.

Septic screen

- Blood cultures from intravascular catheters and a peripheral vein
- Pus samples (better than swabs at identifying organisms)
- Wound swabs
- Sputum or tracheal aspirates
- Urine and faeces.

Antibiotics

β-lactam antibiotics

- All members contain a β-lactam ring structure
- Mode of action is to inhibit cell wall synthesis
- Classification system:
  - Penicillins
  - Cephalosporins
  - Carbapenems.

Allergy and side effects

- Allergic reactions:
  - Anaphylaxis to penicillin (Type I, IgE-mediated reaction) presents with pruritus, flushing, urticaria, angioedema, and hypotension but is rare (1–4/10,000 administrations). All β-lactam antibiotics should be avoided in these patients.
  - Serum sickness—late reaction with fever, rash, adenopathy, and arthritis.
  - 2% of patients with true penicillin allergy (positive skin test) will react after cephalosporin administration. 1% of patients with true penicillin allergy will react to a carbapenem.
  - Dermatological—skin rash, usually maculopapular or morbilliform starting within 2 weeks of starting antibiotic seen in 1–5% of exposed patients.
- Gastrointestinal:
  - Diarrhoea, *C. difficile* infection (as with any antibiotic).
- Hepatobiliary:
  - Cholestatic jaundice—usually flucloxacillin and β-lactamase-resistant penicillins. Ceftriaxone can cause biliary sludging.
- Renal:
  - Interstitial nephritis, glomerulonephritis.
- Central nervous system:
  - Encephalopathy with high-dose treatment, seizures.
- Haematological
  - Haemolytic anaemia, thrombocytopaenia, neutropenia.

Penicillins

Classification

- Benzylpenicillin (also known as Pen G)
- Orally absorbed penicillins (e.g. Pen V)
- Antistaphylococcal penicillins (e.g. meticillin, flucloxacillin)
- Extended-spectrum penicillins (e.g. amoxicillin)
- β-lactamase-resistant penicillins (e.g. co-amoxiclav, piperacillin/tazobactam)

Clinical uses

- Benzylpenicillin is used to treat infections due to *Streptococcus pyogenes* (e.g. cellulitis, necrotizing fasciitis), *Streptococcus agalactiae* and *Streptococcus pneumoniae* (if susceptible to penicillin).
- Penicillin V is used for mild infections due to these agents, primarily pharyngitis ('Strep throat') and for *S. pneumoniae* prophylaxis in asplenic patients.
- Flucloxacillin is the standard antibiotic therapy for meticillin-sensitive *Staphylococcus aureus* (MSSA) infections, as well as empirical therapy for skin and soft tissue infections.
- Amoxicillin is used to treat infections caused by most enterococci and some susceptible Gram-negative organisms such as *Escherichia coli*. Due to advantages in oral absorption over penicillin V, amoxicillin is often used to treat community-acquired pneumonia in order to target *S. pneumoniae* which is the most common cause.
- β-lactamase-resistant penicillins are used to target organisms that produce β-lactamase enzymes which destroy the β-lactam ring of Pen V, Pen G and amoxicillin. Co-amoxiclav is a combination of clavulanic acid, which is a potent inhibitor of many β-lactamases and amoxicillin. Co-amoxiclav is often used to treat HAIs such as pneumonia where resistance is often more of an issue. Tazobactam is similar in potency to clavulanic acid, but when combined with piperacillin (Tazocin®), results in broad-spectrum Gram-positive and Gram-negative activity including against *Pseudomonas aeruginosa*.

Cephalosporins

Classification

- 1st generation—usually used for treatment of simple urinary tract infection, e.g. cephalexin.
- 2nd generation—enhanced Gram-negative activity, e.g. cefuroxime.
- 3rd generation—further enhancement of Gram-negative cover, e.g. cefotaxime, ceftriaxone, and ceftazidime (active against *P. aeruginosa*).
- 4th generation—improved spectrum of activity including *P. aeruginosa*, e.g. cefepime.
- 5th generation—new agents as yet not widely available, e.g. ceftobiprole with activity against MRSA.

Clinical uses

- Alternatives exist for most clinical infection syndromes, therefore cephalosporin use has fallen significantly in recent years.

- Cefuroxime is still used as part of surgical prophylaxis in some hospitals, although there is a drive to change this to flucloxacillin ±gentamicin.
- Ceftriaxone is still the preferred agent in the treatment of bacterial meningitis; however, it is also being used as part of outpatient antibiotic therapy (OPAT) services.
- Ceftazidime is an effective agent for treatment of *P. aeruginosa* infections.

Carbapenems
- Broad-spectrum antibiotics with activity against Gram-positive, Gram-negative, and anaerobic bacteria.

Classification
- Imipenem—first licensed carbapenem, although associated with CNS toxicity.
- Ertapenem—once-daily carbapenem with no activity against *P. aeruginosa* but active against other Gram-negative organisms and anaerobes.
- Meropenem—activity against *P. aeruginosa* and the most commonly used carbapenem, with approval to treat CNS infection as well.

Clinical uses
- Used to treat a wide variety of severe infections such as intra-abdominal sepsis, complicated urinary tract infection, pneumonia, and bacteraemia.
- Meropenem is licensed for treatment of bacterial meningitis.

Glycopeptides
Vancomycin and teicoplanin inhibit cell wall synthesis and are bactericidal against most Gram-positive bacteria:
- Glycopeptides are not absorbed when given orally, therefore they *must* be given by IV infusion for all suspected or proven infections apart from CDI.

Clinical uses
- Continuous ambulatory peritoneal dialysis peritonitis
- Catheter-related bloodstream infection
- Oral vancomycin is the second-line treatment for CDI that is not responding to metronidazole.

Side effects
- Are more common with vancomycin than with teicoplanin.
- Red man syndrome—infusion-related histamine-mediated flushing during or immediately following rapid infusion.
- 5–15% develop a decline in renal function; monitor drug levels.
- 20–30% of patients develop nephrotoxicity when vancomycin is given with an aminoglycoside such as gentamicin.
- Ototoxicity is rare.

Aminoglycosides

- Gentamicin is the most commonly used aminoglycoside in UK, with others, such as amikacin and tobramycin, reserved for specific situations or in the treatment of gentamicin-resistant organisms.
- Aminoglycosides inhibit bacterial protein synthesis and are bactericidal against Gram-negative and some Gram-positive organisms.
- Clinical uses:
  - Surgical prophylaxis in combination with a β-lactam or glycopeptide antibiotic.
  - Empirical therapy of severe infections such as complicated urinary sepsis, intra-abdominal sepsis, and neutropenic sepsis often in combination with other agents.
  - Targeted therapy against numerous Gram-negative organisms such as *E. coli* and *P. aeruginosa*, as well as in combination with a β-lactam or glycopeptide antibiotic in order to treat staphylococcal or streptococcal infection.
  - Topical gentamicin used in treatment of eye and ear infections. Aerosolized tobramycin used in CF patients.

Allergy and side effects

- Nephrotoxicity—incidence estimated at 10–20%, although toxicity is reversible.
- Ototoxicity may result in vestibular or cochlear damage which may lead to irreversible hearing loss.
- Neuromuscular blockade—aminoglycosides contraindicated in myasthenia gravis.
- If patients need to continue therapy beyond 48 hours, trough drug levels should be monitored.

Quinolones

- Quinolones inhibit bacterial nucleic acid synthesis and are bactericidal against both Gram-positive and Gram-negative organisms.

Classification

- Ciprofloxacin is the most commonly used quinolone in UK, and has potent Gram-negative activity, including *P. aeruginosa* and some activity against staphylococci but little activity against *Streptococcus pneumoniae*. Ciprofloxacin also has some activity against *Legionella pneumophila, Mycoplasma pneumoniae* and *Chlamydophila pneumoniae*.
- Norfloxacin and ofloxacin have a similar antimicrobial spectrum to ciprofloxacin.
- Moxifloxacin and levofloxacin have Gram-negative coverage similar to that of ciprofloxacin; however, they are less active against *P. aeruginosa*. Both moxifloxacin and levofloxacin are more active against *S. pneumoniae, Legionella pneumophila, Mycoplasma pneumoniae*, and *Chlamydophila pneumoniae* when compared to ciprofloxacin.

Clinical uses

- Extensive, especially in patients with true penicillin allergy.
- Ciprofloxacin used in treatment of pyelonephritis, urinary tract infection, pneumonia, bone and joint infection, pseudomonal infection, and salmonella infection.

- Ofloxacin is used in treatment of prostatitis, gonorrhoeae, and pelvic inflammatory disease.
- Levofloxacin and moxifloxacin are used second-line for treatment of community-acquired pneumonia, as well as in the treatment of tuberculosis.

Allergy and side effects
- GI symptoms are most common and quinolones have been implicated in several *C. difficile* outbreaks worldwide.
- CNS symptoms such as headache and dizziness have been reported in up to 11% of patients. Quinolones may induce seizures in patients with epilepsy and should be avoided.
- Rash occurs in 0.4–2.2% of patients.
- Tendon rupture has been reported in adults.
- Arthropathy was seen in juvenile animal studies but has yet to be seen in humans.
- QT prolongation has been observed, especially with newer agents.

Macrolides
- These antibiotics inhibit bacterial protein synthesis.

Classification
- Erythromycin and clarithromycin have similar antimicrobial spectrum as penicillin and are commonly used in patients labelled penicillin allergic. They are active against some staphylococci, specifically MSSA, and most streptococci. They are also active against the agents causing atypical pneumonia, namely *Legionella pneumophila*, *Mycoplasma pneumoniae*, and *Chlamydophila pneumoniae*.
- Azithromycin has greater Gram-negative activity than erythromycin and can be given as a single dose to treat chlamydial infections.

Clinical uses
- Used to treat community-acquired pneumonia, usually in combination with a β-lactam.
- Also used to treat severe campylobacter gastroenteritis.
- Clarithromycin used in *Helicobacter pylori* eradication.

Allergy and side effects
- GI symptoms common with erythromycin, but less so with other macrolides, cholestatic jaundice.
- QT prolongation has been seen with all macrolides.
- Skin rash.

Further reading

Fishman NO. Antimicrobial management and cost containment. In Mandell GE, Bennet JE, Dolin R (eds), *Principles and Practice of Infectious Diseases* (5th edn, pp. 539–46). London: Churchill Livingstone; 2000.

Vincent JL, Rello J, Marshall J, Silva E, Anzueto A, Martin CD, et al. EPIC II Group: International study of the prevalence and outcomes of infection in intensive care units. *JAMA* 2009;302(21):2323–9.

Bedside echocardiography

Introduction

Bedside echocardiography has developed into a valuable diagnostic and monitoring tool. Within the CICU it is used to assist the intensivist in making rapid diagnoses and initiating appropriate interventions.

Indications

- Diagnosis of haemodynamic instability:
  - Cardiac failure
  - MI
  - PE
  - Pericardial effusions
  - Cardiac tamponade
  - Valvular problems
  - Cardiac arrest
- Estimation of volume status
- Monitoring the effects of interventions
- LV assessment:
  - Size
  - Degree of filling
  - Contractility
  - Regional wall-motion abnormalities
- RV assessment:
  - Size
  - Degree of filling
  - Contractility
- Evaluation of pyrexia of unknown origin
- Assessment of endocarditis
- Assessment of failure to wean
- Aid to placement of ECMO cannula/IABP.

Transthoracic or transoesophageal echocardiography?

Echocardiographic images of the heart can be obtained through the chest wall (transthoracic echocardiography (TTE)) or from the oesophagus (transoesophageal echocardiography (TOE)). TTE is a safe, non-invasive technique that can be rapidly performed in awake and sedated patients. It is the preferred technique in the critical care environment. However, if a TTE examination provides unsatisfactory views, it may be necessary to perform a TOE examination of the heart. TOE, a semi-invasive technique, is preferable to TTE in a number of specific situations: a detailed interrogation of the mitral valve (including prosthetic valves), assessment of the left atrial appendage for clot formation, assessment of vegetations associated with endocarditis, and suspected aortic dissection.

Use TTE for:

- Assessment of pericardial effusions
- Optimal views of the left ventricular apex
- Optimal views of the left atrium
- Assessment of volume status using the inferior vena cava and subhepatic veins
- Optimal Doppler beam alignment in apical view for aortic, mitral, and tricuspid valves.

Use TOE for:

- Inadequate TTE views (e.g. obesity, chest wall abnormalities, emphysema, IPPV with high levels of positive end expiratory pressure)
- Assessment of structures close to the oesophagus (e.g. left atrial appendage, mitral valve)
- Interrogation of prosthetic mitral valves
- Assessment of vegetations
- Suspected aortic dissection.

Transthoracic echocardiography

Understanding the image

The heart is situated in the anterior mediastinum, with its long axis lying along a line from the right shoulder to the left nipple. When viewed from the front the most anterior structures are the right atrium and right ventricle and the most posterior structure is the left atrium. The ultrasound transducer produces a thin fan-shaped beam that slices through the heart. The slice or image that is achieved depends on the position of the probe on the chest. TTE uses various standard positions (or windows) on the chest in order to assess cardiac structure and function. The images are displayed on a screen with the top of the screen representing the position of the transducer—structures closer to the transducer are seen nearer the top of the screen.

Echocardiography windows

There are three main echocardiography 'windows' in the chest and abdomen that allow ultrasound waves to be transmitted to and reflected from the heart. It is also possible to visualize the lungs (Fig. 32.1).

Subcostal window
- Place the transducer parallel to the skin inferior to the right costal margin and direct the ultrasound beam upwards towards the heart.

Apical window
- Place the transducer over the apex of the heart and direct the ultrasound beam parallel to the long axis of the heart—aim towards the sternum.

Parasternal window
- Place the transducer adjacent to the left sternal margin in the 2nd–4th intercostal space.

Pleural window
- Place the transducer on the lateral thoracic wall.

Preparing the patient

Optimizing the position of the patient will help improve the quality of the images you obtain. Subcostal images are best obtained with the patient lying flat on their back with a relaxed abdomen. For parasternal and apical images, tilting the patient to the left brings the heart closer to the chest wall and improves the images obtained. In addition, abduction of the patient's left arm increases the gap between the ribs and widens the echocardiographic window. The view obtained will change throughout the respiratory cycle. It may be possible to ask spontaneously breathing cooperative patients to hold their breath when the image is at its best. In ventilated patients it may be possible to manipulate the ventilator briefly to obtain the necessary images.

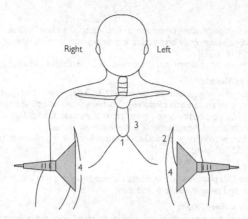

Figure 32.1 Location of the echocar-diography windows. 1: subcostal. 2: apical. 3: parasternal. 4: pleural. Image taken from FATE-card and reproduced with permission from Profes-sor Ph.D. MDSc Erik Sloth. <http://www.usabcd.org> (FATE-app available for free download at App Store and Android Market).

Preparing yourself and the machine

Space is often limited in the critical care bed area, but it is important to position the machine and screen so that you are comfortable whilst scanning. Don't forget to enter the patient's details into the machine and attach ECG leads from the machine to the patient. Identify the 'marker dot' on the probe (this allows the probe to be correctly orientated). Ensure that you have a supply of ultrasound gel and paper towels to clean up the gel at the end. Dim the lights if possible.

With your dominant hand, hold the probe between your thumb and first and second fingers. Ensure there is sufficient ultrasound gel and then apply gentle pressure through the probe to obtain an image. When scanning rest your wrist on the chest wall to prevent the probe from slipping. It is important to learn how small movements of your wrist and probe can alter the image. The probe can rotate, tilt, and slide in order to achieve the desired image. Always scanning from the same position maximizes the benefits of these 'learned movements'. Remember that the image quality may be improved by moving the position of the probe or the position of the patient.

Echo modes

A variety of ultrasound techniques are employed in order to fully assess the heart's structure and function. These include two-dimensional (2D), Motion or M-mode, and Doppler (continuous wave Doppler (CWD), pulsed wave Doppler (PWD), and colour flow mapping (CFM)).

2D Echo

- A succession of slices taken over a cross-section of tissue. When displayed sequentially on a screen it provides 'real-time' imaging of the heart (Fig. 32.2).
- Use to assess anatomy and movement of the ventricles and valves.

Motion or M-mode

- Images of a single slice taken over time (Fig. 32.3). This allows highly accurate measurements of moving structures. The ultrasound beam should be perpendicular to the structure of interest. Computer software allows measurements to be made and stored.
- Use for measurement of cardiac dimensions and timing of events (e.g. diastolic collapse).

Doppler Echo

Uses the Doppler principle to detect the velocity of red blood cells moving towards and away from the transducer.

Continuous wave Doppler

- Measures the maximum blood velocity detected along the length of the ultrasound beam. Cannot therefore localize the exact position of the flow disturbance.
- The calculated velocity is displayed on a velocity/time graph with blood flow towards the transducer displayed above the baseline and flow away displayed below the baseline (Fig. 32.4).
- Can measure high velocities.
- Use to assess valvular stenosis, valvular regurgitation, and the velocity of flow across intracardiac shunts.

Pulsed wave Doppler

- Measures the blood velocity in a specific sample volume (e.g. in the left ventricular outflow tract (LVOT)). The position of the sample volume is selected by the operator.
- The calculated velocity is displayed on a velocity/time graph with blood flow towards the transducer displayed above the baseline and flow away displayed below the baseline (Fig. 32.5).
- Is only accurate below velocities of 2m/s.
- Use for stroke volume and cardiac output calculations.

Colour flow mapping

- Measures blood velocity and direction at several points within a set area.
- The CFM is superimposed on the 2D image. Blood velocities away from the transducer are coloured blue and velocities towards the transducer coloured red (BART: Blue Away Red Towards) (Fig. 32.6). Higher velocities are represented by lighter shades of red or blue. If velocities exceed the processing ability of CFM colour reversal (aliasing) will occur.
- Use for assessing regurgitation and shunts.

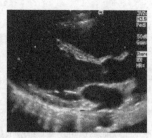

Figure 32.2 Example of 2D Echo.

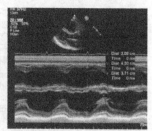

Figure 32.3 Example of M-mode Echo.

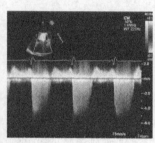

Figure 32.4 Example of CWD.

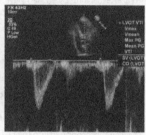

Figure 32.5 Example of PWD.

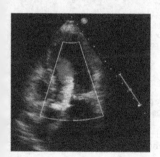

Figure 32.6 Example of CFM.

Abbreviated scanning protocols

A full standard TTE examination involves a series of images and measurements and may take up to 20 minutes. An abbreviated echocardiography examination performed by non-cardiologists has been shown to be both feasible in the critical care environment and contribute significantly to patient management. Whilst cardiologists provide an invaluable service for routine and comprehensive echocardiography, there is a need for a 24 hour a day service for critically ill, haemodynamically unstable patients. The ability to reassess the patient after an intervention is essential. There is therefore a need for an intensivist-led abbreviated echocardiography examination.

Focus-assessed transthoracic echocardiography (FATE)

Within the general intensive care population, TTE performed by trained intensivists, has been shown to provide diagnostic images in 91% of spontaneously breathing and 84% of mechanically ventilated patients and directly change management in >50% of studies.

One abbreviated echocardiographic examination is the FATE protocol. It has been shown to provide one or more useful images of the heart, allowing clinical decision-making, in 97% of patients.

The FATE assessment incorporates the following five views:
- Parasternal long-axis (LAX) view
- Parasternal short-axis (SAX) view
- Apical view
- Subcostal view
- Pleural view.

The aims of the FATE protocol are to:
- Exclude obvious pathology
- Assess contractility
- Assess wall thickness and dimensions of the chambers
- Visualize the pleura on both sides
- Relate the information to the clinical context.

The views incorporated into the FATE assessment will be discussed in detail over the following pages.

Further reading

Jensen MB, Sloth E, Larsen KM, Schmidt MB. Transthoracic echocardiography for cardiopulmonary monitoring in intensive care. *Eur J Anaesthesiol* 2004;21:700–7.

Orme RML'E, Oram MP, McKinstry CE. Impact of echocardiography on patient management in the intensive care unit: an audit of district general hospital practice. *B J Anaesthes* 2009;102(3):340–4.

Parasternal long axis

Obtaining the view

- Patient tilted towards their left.
- Marker dot orientated towards the patient's right shoulder.
- Place the transducer adjacent to the left sternal margin the 2nd–4th intercostal space.
- The mitral and aortic valves should be in the middle of the image with the left ventricular walls lying horizontally across the screen.

Image explained (Fig. 32.7)

- Right ventricle: chamber closest to the transducer at the top of the screen. Use M-mode to measure size.
- Aortic valve: assess leaflet movement and use CFM to identify regurgitation.
- Aortic root and ascending aorta: measure the dimensions of the LVOT, sinuses of Valsalva, sinotubular junction, and ascending aorta.

- Mitral valve: anterior leaflet (closest to transducer) and posterior leaflets seen. assess leaflet movement and use CFM to identify regurgitation.
- Left ventricle: septal and posterior walls. Use M-mode to measure size, function, and wall thickness.
- Left atrium: use M-mode to measure size.
- Descending aorta: circular structure posterior to the left atrium.
- Pericardial effusions: may be identified in front of the right ventricle or behind the left ventricle. Measure using M-mode.

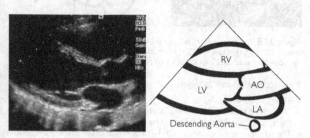

Figure 32.7 Parasternal long-axis view: image and line diagram. RV, right ventricle; LV, left ventricle; AO, ascending aorta; LA, left atrium.

Parasternal short axis (aortic)

Obtaining the view

- Centre the parasternal long axis view on the aortic valve and rotate the transducer clockwise through 90° until the heart is seen in transverse section. By directing the ultrasound beam from the patient's right shoulder to left flank, serial short-axis (transverse) slices through the heart from the base to apex can be obtained.
- Marker dot now orientated towards the patient's left shoulder.
- The aortic valve should appear in the centre of the screen with all three of its cusps visible. The tricuspid and pulmonary valves are seen on the left and right of the screen respectively.

Image explained (Fig. 32.8)

- Right ventricle: the most anterior chamber (nearest the transducer) that curves around the aortic valve.
- Aortic valve: seen in the centre of the screen with a 'Mercedes Benz logo' appearance. Assess leaflet movement and use CFM to identify regurgitation.
- Tricuspid valve: seen to the left of the screen. Assess leaflet movement and use CFM to identify regurgitation. Estimate pulmonary artery pressure using CWD.
- Pulmonary valve: seen to the right of the screen. Assess leaflet movement and use CFM to identify regurgitation. Use CWD to identify outflow obstruction.

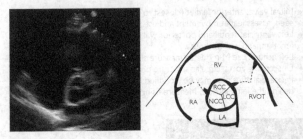

Figure 32.8 Parasternal short-axis (aortic) view: image and line diagram. RA, right atrium; RV, right ventricle; RVOT, right ventricular outflow tract; LA, left atrium; RCC, right coronary cusp; LCC, left coronary cusp; NCC, non-coronary cusp.

Parasternal short axis (mitral)

Obtaining the view

- From the parasternal short-axis aortic view, tilt the transducer towards the apex of the heart/left flank. This is a very small movement.
- The left ventricle should be round and symmetrical with the 'fish mouth' view of the mitral valve visible.

Image explained (Fig. 32.9)

- Mitral valve: anterior (closest to the transducer) and posterior leaflets clearly seen. Assess leaflet movement. Assess stenosis by tracing the valve area (planimetry) and use CFM to identify regurgitation.

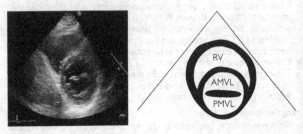

Figure 32.9 Parasternal short-axis (mitral) view: image and line diagram. RV, right ventricle; AMVL, anterior mitral valve leaflet; PMVL, posterior mitral valve leaflet.

Parasternal short axis (mid-papillary)

Obtaining the view

- From the parasternal short-axis mitral view, tilt the transducer a little more towards the apex of the heart (left flank) until the bodies of the papillary muscles come into view.
- The left ventricle should be round and symmetrical and the bodies of both papillary muscles seen.

Image explained (Fig. 32.10)

- Left ventricle: septal, anterior, lateral, and inferior walls seen. Use M-mode to measure size and wall thickness. Can assess global and regional LV function.
- Right ventricle: use M-mode to measure size and look for any diastolic collapse.

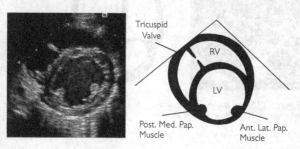

Figure 32.10 Parasternal SAX view (mid papillary): image and line diagram. RV, right ventricle; LV, left ventricle.

Apical 4-chamber

Obtaining the view

- Place the transducer over the apex of the heart and direct the ultrasound beam parallel to the long axis of the heart.
- Marker dot orientated towards the patient's left flank.
- All four chambers and the mitral and tricuspid valves should be seen. The ventricular septum should lie vertically down the centre of the screen.

Image explained (Fig. 32.11)

Left-sided chambers are seen to the right of the screen.

- Left ventricle: septal, apical, and lateral walls seen. Can assess global and regional LV function.
- Right ventricle: assess size (compare with left) and function.
- Atria: right and left atria and intra-atrial septum are seen. Can assess atrial volumes.
- Mitral valve: anterior and posterior mitral valve leaflets seen. Assess leaflet movement. Assess stenosis by using CWD to calculate the pressure half time. Use CFM to identify regurgitation.
- Tricuspid valve: lateral and septal leaflets seen. Assess leaflet movement and use CFM to identify regurgitation. Estimate pulmonary artery pressure using CWD.

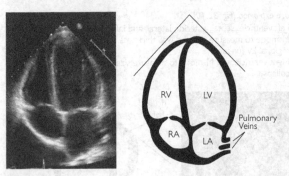

Figure 32.11 Apical 4-chamber view: image and line diagram. RV, right ventricle; LV, left ventricle; RA, right atrium; LA left atrium.

Apical 5-chamber

Obtaining the view

- From the apical 4-chamber view, angle the transducer anteriorly towards the chest wall until the '5th chamber' (the LVOT) comes into view.

Image explained (Fig. 32.12)

- Aortic valve: assess leaflet movement and use CFM to identify regurgitation. Assess stenosis by using CWD to determine the peak velocity/peak gradient.
- LVOT: use PWD to calculate the velocity–time integral (VTI) of the LVOT, which can be used, along with the cross-sectional area of the LVOT, to calculate cardiac output.

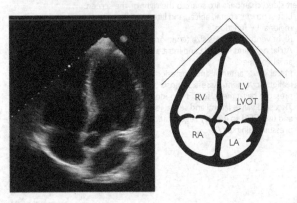

Figure 32.12 Apical 5-chamber view: image and line diagram. RV, right ventricle; LV, left ventricle; RA, right atrium; LA, left atrium; LVOT, left ventricular outflow tract.

Subcostal

Obtaining the view

- Increase the depth of the image.
- Patient lying flat on their back, abdomen relaxed, and knees bent.
- Hold the probe in the palm of your hand. Place the transducer parallel to the skin inferior to the right costal margin and direct the ultrasound beam under the ribs, towards the heart. Gentle downwards pressure may be needed.
- Marker dot orientated towards the patient's left shoulder.
- All four chambers and the mitral and tricuspid valves should be seen. The septa should lie horizontally across the screen.

Image explained (Fig. 32.13)

Good view to assess right-sided chambers (as they lie closest to the transducer) and pericardial effusions. This is an alternative view if unable to obtain parasternal views.

- Liver: top left of the image. Freely transmits ultrasound waves.
- Diaphragm: hyperechoic linear structure between the liver and the right heart that moves with respiration.
- Right ventricle: adjacent to the diaphragm. Free wall and septum seen. Compare size with left and assess function. Use M-mode to measure size and wall thickness. Assess intra-ventricular septum for defects using CFM.
- Right atrium: assess intra-atrial septum for defects using CFM. Use M-mode to measure size.
- Tricuspid valve: assess leaflet movement and use CFM to identify regurgitation.
- Left ventricle: septal and lateral walls seen.
- Left atrium: use M-mode to measure size.
- Mitral valve: assess leaflet movement.
- Pericardium: assess size and depth of any effusions.

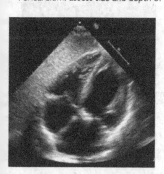
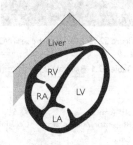

Figure 32.13 Subcostal view: image and line diagram. RV, right ventricle; LV, left ventricle; RA, right atrium; LA, left atrium.

Inferior vena cava

Obtaining the view

- From the subcostal view rotate the transducer anticlockwise whilst keeping the right atrium in view.
- The inferior vena cava (IVC) appears as a tubular structure that empties into the right atrium.

Image explained (Figs 32.14 and 32.15)

- IVC: measure the diameter and any changes associated with respiration in order to estimate right atrial pressure (Table 32.1).

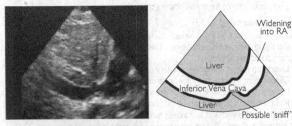

Figure 32.14 IVC view: image and line diagram. RA, right atrium.

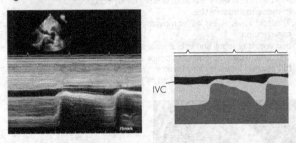

Figure 32.15 Example of change in IVC diameter with 'sniffing': image and line diagram.

Table 32.1 Right atrial pressure (mmHg)

	0–5	5–10	10–15	15–20	>20
IVC					
Size (cm)	<1.5	1.5–2.5	1.5–2.5	>2.5	>2.5
Respiratory/sniff variation	Collapse	↓>50%	↓<50%	↓<50%	No change
Other					
RA size	Normal	Normal	↑	↑↑	↑↑

IVC, inferior vena cava; RA, right atrium.

Pleural

Obtaining the view

- Place the transducer on the lateral thoracic wall in the mid axillary line.
- Marker dot orientated towards the patient's axilla.
- Caudal structures seen to the left of the screen. Identify the diagram, liver, and lung tissue.

Image explained (Fig. 32.16)

- Diaphragm: a bright line that curves across the image and moves with respiration.
- Liver/spleen: seen on the left of the image adjacent to the diaphragm.
- Lung tissue: seen on the right of the image.
- Pleural effusion: appears as a hypoechoic (dark) area.

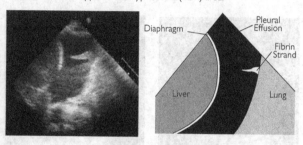

Figure 32.16 Pleural view with effusion: image and line diagram.

Investigating hypotension

Unexplained hypotension in the CICU is usually secondary to hypovolaemia, vasodilatation, or cardiac failure. Bedside echocardiography can be used to help differentiate between these possible causes.

Hypovolaemia or vasodilatation?

Hypovolaemia

Hypovolaemia results in reduced left ventricular filling. The volume/area/diameter (surrogates for left ventricular filling) of the left ventricle at end diastole and end systole will therefore be noticeably reduced. Starting from smaller than normal at end diastole, the left ventricle contracts until the papillary muscles are close to meeting—kissing papillary muscles.

Vasodilatation

Vasodilatation results in ↓ peripheral vascular resistance and therefore ↑ stroke volumes. End-diastolic left ventricular volume remains constant but end systolic volumes are reduced. Starting from normal size at end diastole, the left ventricle contracts until the papillary muscles are close to meeting.

- Obtain short-axis images of the left ventricle (parasternal SAX view).
- Measure the internal diameter (LVID)/trace the internal circumference of the left ventricle in end diastole (LVIDd) and end systole (LVIDs) (Figs 32.17, 32.18, 32.19, and 32.20).

Cardiac failure

Hypotension may be due to the:
- Left ventricle:
  - Global dysfunction
  - Regional dysfunction
  - LV outflow obstruction (systolic anterior motion of the mitral valve)
- Right ventricle:
  - Systolic dysfunction
  - RV outflow tract obstruction (PE)
- Pericardium:
  - Fluid (tamponade)
  - Thickening (constrictive pericarditis).

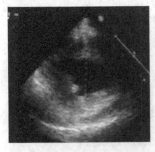

Figure 32.17 Parasternal SAX view. End diastole. LVIDd = 2.66cm.

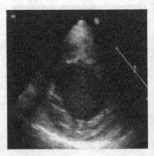

Figure 32.18 Parasternal SAX view. End diastole. LVIDd = 3.89cm.

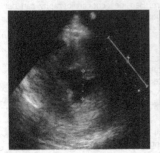

Figure 32.19 Parasternal SAX view. End systole LVIDs = 1.61cm.

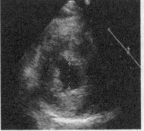

Figure 32.20 Parasternal SAX view. End systole LVIDs = 1.46cm.

Assessment of the left ventricle

- Eye ball test
- Dimensions and fractional shortening/ejection fraction
- Measurement of CO.

Eyeball test

Use the parasternal short axis mid papillary view to obtain an overall picture of the heart's function. Standardize the depth of the image to facilitate comparison and pattern recognition. See Fig. 32.21.

Is the heart empty or full?
- Do the papillary muscles touch at end systole in the parasternal SAX view?
- Assess the IVC in the subcostal view.
- Assess RA size.

Is the heart contracting well?
- Does it appear to move in a smooth or jerky manner?

Is there a regional wall-motion abnormality?
- Look at each segment in turn. Placing a finger in the centre of the image may help identify an abnormally contracting segment.
- Segments may be normal, hypokinetic, akinetic, or move paradoxically (dyskinetic).

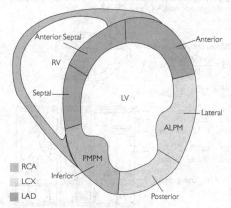

Figure 32.21 Parasternal short axis diagram illustrating coronary territories. RV, right ventricle; LV, left ventricle; ALPM, anterolateral papillary muscle; PMPM, posteromedial papillary muscle; RCA, right coronary artery; LCX, left circumflex artery; LAD, left anterior descending. Reproduced with kind permission from *Practical Perioperative Transoesophageal Echocardiography*, David Sidebotham, Alan Merry, Malcolm Legget, 2003, Figure 17.7, p. 288, Copyright the authors.

Calculating fractional shortening and ejection fraction

M-mode

Use M-mode through the base of the heart (tips of the mitral valve leaflets) in the parasternal LAX view (Figs 32.22 and 32.23). Measure the left ventricular size at end diastole (timed with the R wave on the ECG) and at end systole (timed with the T wave on the ECG). The inbuilt software on the machine will then estimate the fractional shortening and ejection fraction.

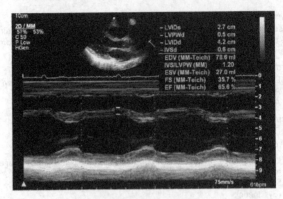

Figure 32.22 Example of calculation of fractional shortening and ejection fraction using M-mode (parasternal LAX view).

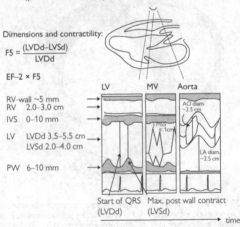

Figure 32.23 Line diagram of parasternal long-axis M-mode. Image taken from FATE-card and reproduced with permission from Professor Ph.D. MDSc Erik Sloth. <http://www.usabcd.org> (FATE-app available for free download at App Store and Android Market).

Simpson's method

Simpson's method divides the left ventricle into a series of discs providing a 3D estimation of LV volume (Fig. 32.24). Using the inbuilt software, estimation of end-diastolic and end-systolic LV volumes facilitates estimation of the LV ejection fraction. This method can be made more accurate by repeating the process in another plane (apical 2-chamber) and taking the average of the values obtained.

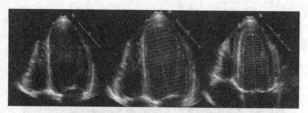

Figure 32.24 Simpson's method for estimation of ejection fraction. Obtain an apical 4-chamber view. Ensure that the endocardial border of the LV is clearly defined and that the ventricle is not foreshortened (ensure the apex is identified: it is fixed and doesn't move towards the base during systole). Zoom in on the left ventricle and then record a loop. At end diastole (R wave on ECG), trace the endocardial border and note the calculated end diastolic volume (EDV). Scroll to end systole (T wave on ECG), trace the endocardial border and note the end systolic volume (ESV). The ejection fraction can then be calculated:

$$\text{Ejection fraction}(\%) = \frac{\text{EDV} - \text{ESV}}{\text{EDV}} \times 100$$

Measuring cardiac output

Consider the flow in the LVOT. The volume of blood flowing through the LVOT over a given time period is the product of the cross-sectional area of the LVOT and the VTI:

$$\text{Stoke volume}_{\text{LVOT}} = \text{cross-sectional area}_{\text{LVOT}} \times \text{VTI}_{\text{LVOT}}$$

Cross-sectional area of the LVOT

- Area of a circle = $\pi \times \text{radius}^2$.
- Measure the diameter of the LVOT in the parasternal LAX view (radius=½ diameter). Ensure this is accurate as the value (and therefore any error) is being squared.

Velocity time integral of LVOT

- Apical 5-chamber view.
- Use PWD with the sample chamber situated in the LVOT.
- On the resulting velocity–time graph, trace the outline of the velocity to calculate the VTI.

The volume through the LVOT can be used to calculate cardiac output:

$$\text{cardiac output} = \text{volume}_{\text{LVOT}} \times \text{heart rate}$$

See Fig. 32.25 and Table 32.2.

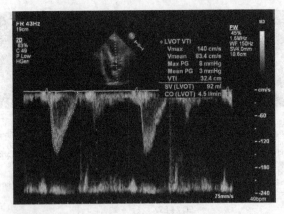

Figure 32.25 PWD with sample chamber in LVOT. VTI calculated.

Table 32.2 Left ventricular dimensions and function

	Normal	Mild	Moderate	Severe
LV wall thickness				
IVSd/PWd (cm)	0.6–1.2	1.3–1.5	1.6–1.9	≥2
LV dimensions, women				
LVIDd (cm)	3.9–5.3	5.4–5.7	5.8–6.1	≥6.2
LVIDd/BSA (cm/m^2)	2.4–3.2	3.3–3.4	3.5–3.7	≥3.8
LV dimensions, men				
LVIDd (cm)	4.2–5.9	6.0–6.3	6.4–6.8	≥6.9
LVIDd/BSA (cm/m^2)	2.2–3.1	3.2–3.4	3.5–3.6	≥3.7
LV volume, women				
LV diastolic volume (mL)	56–104	105–117	118–130	≥131
LV systolic volume (mL)	19–49	50–59	60–69	≥70
LV volume, men				
LV diastolic volume (mL)	67–155	156–178	179–201	≥202
LV systolic volume (mL)	22–58	59–70	71–82	≥83
LV volume index				
LV diastolic volume/BSA (mL/m^2)	35–75	76–86	87–96	≥97
LV systolic volume/BSA (mL/m^2)	12–30	31–36	37–42	≥43

(Continued)

Table 32.2 (Continued)

	Normal	Mild	Moderate	Severe
LV function				
Fractional shortening (%)	25–43	20–24	15–19	<15
EF (Simpson's method) (%)	≥55	45–54	36–44	≤35
LA size, women				
LA diameter (cm)	2.7–3.8	3.9–4.2	4.3–4.6	≥4.7
LA volume (mL)	22–52	53–62	63–72	≥73
LA size, men				
LA diameter (cm)	3.0–4.0	4.1–4.6	4.7–5.2	≥5.3
LA volume (mL)	18–58	59–68	69–78	≥79
LA size, index				
LA diameter (cm/m²)	1.5–2.3	2.4–2.6	2.7–2.9	≥3.0
LA volume (mL/m²)	16–28	29–33	34–39	≥40

BSA, body surface area; EF, ejection fraction; IVSd, intraventricular septum diameter; LA, left atrium; LV, left ventricle; PWd, posterior wall diameter; LVIDd, left ventricular internal diameter diastole. Reproduced from the *Journal of the American Society of Echocardiography*, 18, 12, Lang, M., et al. Recommendations for Chamber Quantification: A Report from the American Society of Echocardiography's Guidelines and Standards Committee and the Chamber Quantification Writing Group, Developed in Conjunction with the European Association of Echocardiography, a Branch of the European Society of Cardiology, pp. 1440–1463, Copyright 2005, with permission from American Society of Echocardiography and Elsevier.

Assessment of the right ventricle

- Eye ball test
- Dimensions and fractional area change
- Estimating pulmonary artery pressure.

See Table 32.3.

Eyeball test

In the apical 4-chamber view compare the right ventricle with the left ventricle.

- The right ventricular area should be smaller than (usually 2/3) the area of the left ventricle and the cardiac apex formed solely by the left ventricle.
- Equally sized ventricles suggest a moderately dilated right ventricle.
- If the right is larger than the left and forms the cardiac apex, then the right ventricle is severely dilated.

Right ventricular dimensions

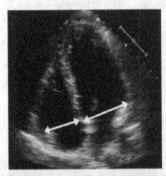

Figure 32.26 Basal diameter RV. Apical 4-chamber view. Normal diameter 2–2.8 cm

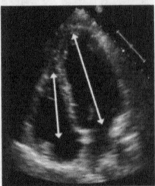

Figure 32.27 RV length. Apical 4-chamber view. Normal length 7.1–7.9cm.

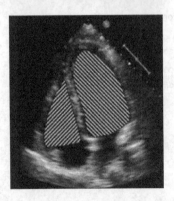

Figure 32.28 RV area. Apical 4-chamber view. Estimate RV function by measuring area in systole and diastole to calculate fractional area change.

Table 32.3 Right ventricular dimensions and function

	Normal	Mild	Moderate	Severe
RV dimensions (apical 4 chamber)				
Basal RV diameter (cm)	2.0–2.8	2.9–3.3	3.4–3.8	≥3.9
Base to apex length (cm)	7.1–7.9	8.0–8.5	8.6–9.1	≥9.2
PA diameter (parasternal SAX)				
Main PA (cm)	1.5–2.1	2.2–2.5	2.6–2.9	≥3.0
RV area				
RV diastolic area (cm^2)	11–28	29–32	33–37	≥38
RV systolic area (cm^2)	7.5–16	17–19	20–22	≥23
RV function				
Fractional area change (%)	32–60	25–31	18–24	≤17

RV, right ventricle; PA pulmonary artery. Reproduced from the *Journal of the American Society of Echocardiography*, 18, 12, Lang, M., et al. Recommendations for Chamber Quantification: A Report from the American Society of Echocardiography's Guidelines and Standards Committee and the Chamber Quantification Writing Group, Developed in Conjunction with the European Association of Echocardiography, a Branch of the European Society of Cardiology, pp. 1440–1463, Copyright 2005, with permission from American Society of Echocardiography and Elsevier.

Estimating pulmonary artery pressure

• Use an apical 4-chamber or parasternal SAX view with a visible jet of tricuspid regurgitation.
• Align CWD through the tricuspid valve regurgitation.
• Measure the peak velocity.
• The tricuspid pressure gradient is calculated from the peak velocity using a modified Bernoulli equation:

$$\text{Pressure gradient} = 4 \times \text{peak velocity}^2$$

• The RV systolic pressure, which is equivalent to pulmonary artery systolic pressure in the absence of pulmonary stenosis, is equal to the sum of the tricuspid pressure gradient and right atrial pressure (CVP).

Normal values

Normal values can be found in the Recommendations for chamber quantification: a report from the American Society of Echocardiography's Guidelines and Standards Committee and the Chamber Quantification Writing Group (see 📖 Further reading, p. 361).

There is also an iPhone application named EchoCalc created by the British Society of Echocardiography.

For some examples of important pathologies see Fig. 32.29.

Further reading

Lang RM, Bierig M, Devereux RB, Flachskampf FA, Foster E, Pellikka PA, *et al*. Recommendations for chamber quantification: a report from the American Society of Echocardiography's Guidelines and Standards Committee and the chamber quantification writing group, developed in conjunction with the European Association of Echocardiography, a branch of the European Society of Cardiology. *J Am Soc Echocardiogr* 2005;18:1140–63.

Important pathology

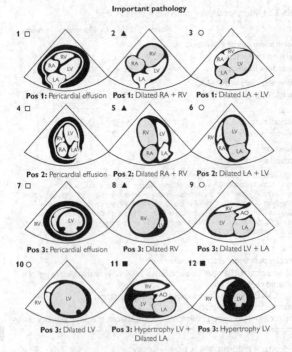

PATHOLOGY TO BE CONSIDERED IN PARTICULAR:

□ Post DC cardiac surgery, following cardiac catheterisation, trauma, renal failure, infection.
▲ Pulmonary embolism, RV infraction, pulmonary hypertension, volume overload.
○ Ischemic heart disease, dilated cardiomyopathy, sepsis, volume overload, aorta insufficiency.
■ Aorta stenosis, arterial hypertension, LV outflow tract obstruction,
  hypertrophic cardiomyopathy, myocardial deposits diseases.

Figure 32.29 Important pathology examples. Image taken from FATE-card and reproduced with permission from Professor Ph.D. MDSc Erik Sloth. <http://www. usabcd.org> (FATE-app available for free download at App Store and Android Market).

Transoesophageal echocardiography

Introduction

This section will provide an overview of the information that can be obtained using TOE in the setting of the CICU. The majority of any echocardiographic examination involves the interpretation of moving images. There are many examples of these available via the Internet which are recommended to the reader.

Risks and precautions

TOE is described as an 'invasive, non-invasive' investigation since there is morbidity and indeed mortality described from its use. As such, safety is of extreme importance and the sonographer must review the patient's history to exclude any contraindication to TOE before undertaking the study. The practice guidelines for perioperative TOE recommend 'that TOE may be used for patients with oral, oesophageal or gastric disease, if the expected benefit outweighs the potential risk, provided the appropriate precautions are applied'. The precautions include considering other imaging techniques (e.g. TTE), asking for an upper GI opinion and perhaps endoscopy, using the smallest available probe, limiting the examination and avoiding unnecessary probe manipulation, and using the most experienced operator.

Prior to the examination consideration must be given to analgesia and sedation, and the monitoring of the patient's vital signs must be delegated to another individual, or the monitors positioned such that the sonographer has a clear view of them during the procedure. This is of particular importance since in the majority of cases TOE is being performed to determine the cause of postoperative haemodynamic instability.

Specific indications for TOE in ICU

- Mitral valve assessment
- Endocarditis
- Embolism of unknown origin
- Unexplained hypoxemia
- Pulmonary thromboembolism
- Aortic dissection.

The standard views

The ASE/SCA practice guidelines suggest 20 standard views to be obtained during a comprehensive TOE exam. There is no generally accepted order in which these views are obtained. Fig. 32.30 shows the views which most commonly provide relevant information in the CICU, and the abnormalities which may be detected.

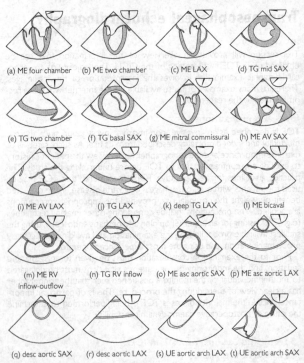

(a) ME four chamber (b) ME two chamber (c) ME LAX (d) TG mid SAX

(e) TG two chamber (f) TG basal SAX (g) ME mitral commissural (h) ME AV SAX

(i) ME AV LAX (j) TG LAX (k) deep TG LAX (l) ME bicaval

(m) ME RV inflow-outflow (n) TG RV inflow (o) ME asc aortic SAX (p) ME asc aortic LAX

(q) desc aortic SAX (r) desc aortic LAX (s) UE aortic arch LAX (t) UE aortic arch SAX

Figure 32.30 The standard views of a comprehensive TOE examination. Reproduced from Shanewise et al. ASE/SCA Guidelines for Performing a Comprehensive Intraoperative Multiplane Transesophageal Echocardiography Examination: Recommendations of the American Society of Echocardiography Council for Intraoperative Echocardiography and the Society of Cardiovascular Anesthesiologists Task Force for Certification in Perioperative Transesophageal Echocardiography. *Anesthesia & Analgesia*, 89, 4, p. 870, copyright 1999, with permission from International Anesthesia Research Society and Wolters Kluwer.

Mitral valve assessment

The mitral valve is immediately close to the oesophagus and TOE provides excellent quality images for the assessment of the mitral valve. This may be essential for determination of the mitral valve morphology and diagnosis of mechanisms of mitral regurgitation. TOE is also invaluable for the assessment of the prosthetic mitral valve or mitral valve repair. The best views are shown in Figs 32.31, 32.32, and 32.33.

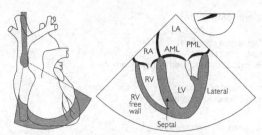

Figure 32.31 Mid oesophageal 4-chamber view (MO 4-chamber). Reproduced with kind permission from *Practical Perioperative Transoesophageal Echocardiography*, David Sidebotham, Alan Merry, Malcolm Legget, 2003, Figure 3.11, p. 40, Copyright the authors.

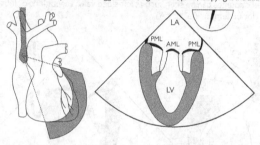

Figure 32.32 Mid oesophageal mitral commissural view (MO mitral commissural) (P3 on left of display, P1 on right, A2 in centre). Reproduced with kind permission from *Practical Perioperative Transoesophageal Echocardiography*, David Sidebotham, Alan Merry, Malcolm Legget, 2003, Figure 3.13, p. 41, Copyright the authors.

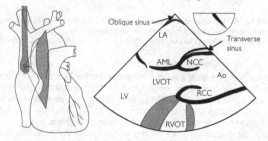

Figure 32.33 Mid oesophageal aortic valve long axis view (MO AV LAX). This view may reveal dynamic LVOT obstruction secondary to systolic anterior motion of the mitral valve (SAM). This uncommon but extremely important cause of hypotension following cardiac surgery is characterized by the anterior leaflet of the mitral valve prolapsing into the LVOT and perhaps even coapting with the interventricular septum which is usually hypertrophied. There is often associated mitral regurgitation and the velocity of this regurgitant jet may reveal that the pressure inside the left ventricle during systole is higher than the systemic blood pressure. Reproduced with kind permission from *Practical Perioperative Transoesophageal Echocardiography*, David Sidebotham, Alan Merry, Malcolm Legget, 2003, Figure 3.5, p. 37, Copyright the authors.

Possible findings in endocarditis

- Vegetations on valves
- Aortic root abscess
- Perforated or destroyed leaflets of any valve
- Dehisced mechanical valve
- Mechanical or bioprosthetic valve dysfunction
- Fistula between chambers.

Embolism of unknown origin

TOE is superior to TTE in the examination of the left atrium and particularly the examination of the left atrial appendage which is a common source of arterial embolism. This is best seen in the MO 2-chamber view. Alternative embolic sources can be seen such as left-sided valve vegetations or intracardiac clot or tumour (LV or LA).

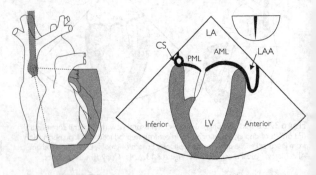

Figure 32.34 Mid oesophageal 2-chamber view (MO 2-chamber). Reproduced with kind permission from *Practical Perioperative Transoesophageal Echocardiography*, David Sidebotham, Alan Merry, Malcolm Legget, 2003, Figure 3.14, p. 41, Copyright the authors.

Unexplained hypoxaemia

Shunt at the intra-atrial level may be revealed either as a result of a patent foramen ovale or an atrial septal defect. Bubble contrast test (injection of agitated saline into the central line) and CFM can help determine the position and direction of any septal defect (Fig. 32.35). This important test to can help to exclude a cardiac cause of hypoxia post cardiac surgery.

Clot compression of the atria may be revealed in this view. Withdrawal of the central line should be considered if examination reveals the tip to be within the right atrium.

Pulmonary thromboembolism

Clot may be seen in the main pulmonary artery in massive pulmonary embolism. This is best seen in the MO ascending aorta SAX view (Fig. 32.36); however, the right main bronchus often partially obscures this view.

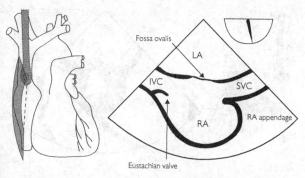

Figure 32.35 Mid oesophageal bicaval view (MO bicaval). Reproduced with kind permission from *Practical Perioperative Transoesophageal Echocardiography*, David Sidebotham, Alan Merry, Malcolm Legget, 2003, Figure 3.9, p. 38, Copyright the authors.

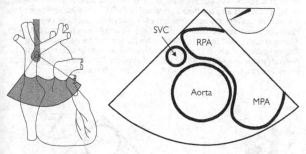

Figure 32.36 Mid oesophageal ascending aortic short-axis view (MO asc. aortic SAX). Reproduced with kind permission from *Practical Perioperative Transoesophageal Echocardiography*, David Sidebotham, Alan Merry, Malcolm Legget, 2003, Figure 3.6, p. 37, Copyright the authors.

Aortic dissection

The assessment of aortic dissection is best done with TOE rather than TTE. Often the patient will have already had a contrast CT scan. A full assessment of the ascending arch and descending aorta should be performed. Classically an endothelial flap will be revealed in the ascending aorta in type 1 dissection. In addition, aortic regurgitation and pericardial haemopericardium may be revealed. In case of dissection into a coronary artery, evidence of a wall-motion abnormality will be present.

In addition to the mid oesophageal aortic valve long-axis view (MO AV LAX) seen earlier (Fig. 32.33) the views in Figs 32.37, 32.38, and 32.39 may be useful.

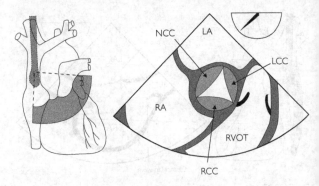

Figure 32.37 Mid oesophageal aortic valve short-axis view (MO AV SAX). The MO AV SAX view is a good starting point since the aortic valve is often easily identified by the Mercedes Benz sign when in the closed position. The left atrium lies closest to the probe and is displayed at the top of the screen. This view offers clear images of the left and right atria and the aortic valve. The RVOT is often less well seen since it is more distant from the transducer and any calcification in the aortic valve will cause ultrasound drop out. Compression of the left or right atria by blood clot which is often enough to lead to post cardiotomy tamponade may be seen in this view. The morphology of the aortic valve is seen. Reproduced with kind permission from *Practical Perioperative Transoesophageal Echocardiography*, David Sidebotham, Alan Merry, Malcolm Legget, 2003, Figure 3.4, p. 37, Copyright the authors.

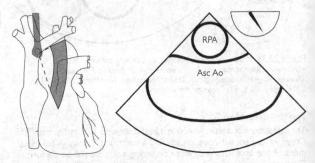

Figure 32.38 Mid oesophageal ascending aortic long-axis view (MO asc. aortic LAX). Reproduced with kind permission from *Practical Perioperative Transoesophageal Echocardiography*, David Sidebotham, Alan Merry, Malcolm Legget, 2003, Figure 3.7, p. 36, Copyright the authors.

Assessment of ventricular function with TOE

Left ventricle

The transgastric mid SAX view is a useful view for the assessment of the LV function. Myocardium supplied by all three main coronary arteries are seen. The view is commonly referred to as the bouncing doughnut view (Fig. 32.39)!

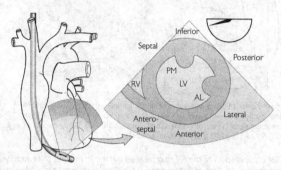

Figure 32.39 Transgastric mid papillary short axis view (TG mid SAX). Reproduced with kind permission from *Practical Perioperative Transoesophageal Echocardiography*, David Sidebotham, Alan Merry, Malcolm Legget, 2003, Figure 3.18, p. 44, Copyright the authors.

Right ventricle

Right ventricular systolic function and dimensions can be assessed in this view (Fig. 32.40). Dilatation of the right ventricle is often associated with tricuspid regurgitation and determination of the peak velocity of the regurgitant jet across the tricuspid valve will provide the right ventricular and therefore the pulmonary artery systolic pressure. (RV systolic pressure = $4 \times V$ max^2 + CVP.) Clot compression of the RV may be seen but it is important to remember that the classic signs of tamponade (associated with pericardial effusion) are often absent in the post cardiac surgery setting with 'regional tamponade' or localized clot collection a common finding.

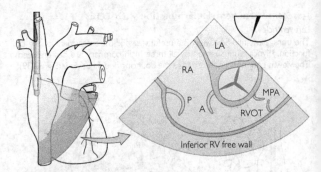

Figure 32.40 Mid oesophageal right ventricular inflow outflow view (MO RV inflow-outflow). Reproduced with kind permission from *Practical Perioperative Transoesophageal Echocardiography*, David Sidebotham, Alan Merry, Malcolm Legget, 2003, Figure 3.8, p. 38, Copyright the authors.

Clot compression of the RV may be seen but it is important to remember that the classic signs of tamponade (associated with pericardial effusion) are often absent in the post cardiac surgery setting with 'regional tamponade' or localized clot collection a common finding.

Index